MANUAL FOR CLINICAL RESEARCH IN BREAST CANCER

5th Edition

EORTC BREAST CANCER GROUP

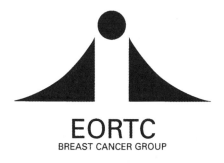

EORTC
BREAST CANCER GROUP

**Published at the occasion of the 4th European Breast Cancer Conference
Hamburg, 16–20 March 2004**

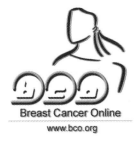

Breast Cancer Online
www.bco.org

The information contained in this book is also available on *Breast Cancer Online*
(www.bco.org) and www.eortc.be/groups.

This publication was supported by an unrestricted educational grant from

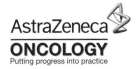

AstraZeneca
ONCOLOGY
Putting progress into practice

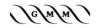

Published by:

Greenwich Medical Media
4th Floor, 137 Euston Road
London, NW1 2AA
UK

Website: www.greenwich-medical.co.uk

ISBN: 1-84110-256-3

1st Edition 1991
2nd Edition 1996
3rd Edition 1998
4th Edition 2000
5th Edition 2004

Every effort has been made to check drug dosages; however, it is still possible that errors have occurred. Furthermore, dosage schedules are constantly being revised and new side effects recognised. For these reasons, the medical practitioner is strongly urged to consult the drug companies' printed instructions before administering any of the drugs mentioned in this book.

The publisher makes no representation, express or implied, with regard to the accuracy of the information contained in this book and cannot accept any legal responsibility or liability for any errors or omissions that may be made.

A catalogue record for this book is available from the British Library.

Typeset by CharonTec Pvt. Ltd, Chennai, India

Printed by Bell and Bain Ltd, Glasgow, Scotland, UK

Acknowledgement

The EORTC Breast Cancer Group wishes to express its sincere gratitude towards the following contributors:

Initial texts submitted by:
L. Beex
J. Borger
P. Cohen
H. de Haes
J. Jassem
J.P. Julien
L. Leunens
M.A. Nooij
R. Paridaens
H. Peterse
M. Piccart
E.J.Th. Rutgers
H. Stewart
R. Sylvester
J. A. van Dongen
E. van Limbergen
A. van Oosterom

Reading Committee 1st Edition:
L. Beex
M. Blichert-Toft
R. Christiaens
T. Delozier
J. Jassem
M.A. Nooij
E.J.Th. Rutgers
H. Stewart
E. van der Schueren

Coordinating editor 1st Edition: K. Vantongelen
Technical preparation 1st Edition: L. Minnen and H. Swinnen
Coordinating editor 2nd Edition (CD-ROM):   J.A. van Dongen
Coordinating editor 3rd Edition (2nd CD-ROM & Print):   J.A. van Dongen

With the assistance of:
L. Beex
A. Geurts-Moespot
H. de Haes
W.J.G.M. Klijn
E. van Limbergen
F. Mignolet
H. Peterse
M. Piccart
E.J.Th. Rutgers
C.G.J. Sweep
R. Sylvester
P. Therasse
K. Vantongelen
C.J.H. van de Velde
C. Vrieling

Coordinating editor 4th Edition (3rd CD-ROM):   M. Blichert-Toft

Additional authors of 4th Edition:
M. Andersson
H. Bartelink
A. Bottomley
J. Kramer
B. Pieters
M. van de Vijver

Coordinating editor 5th edition: J.P. Julien

With the assistance of: J. Jassem and E. Rutgers

Additional authors of 5th Edition:
L. Biganzoli
J. Bonnema
D. Cameron
T. Cufer
V. Distante
C. Van Ongheval
T. van Sprundel
G. van Tienhoven
R. Tollenaar

Technical preparation 5th Edition: J. Remmelzwaal

EORTC Breast Cancer Group

Officers: E. Rutgers, Chairman
         H. Bonnefoi, Secretary
         R. Coleman, Treasurer

EORTC Breast Cancer Group
Avenue E. Mounier, 83, Bte 11
1200 Brussels, Belgium
Phone: + 32 2 774 16 11
Fax: + 32 2 772 35 45
Email: eortc@eortc.be
Website: www.eortc.be

Table of contents

I. Introduction

I.1   Foreword

I.2   Florence statement – Forging the way ahead for more research on and better care in breast cancer

I.3   Brussels statement

I.4   Barcelona Statement – The future of breast cancer research in danger

I.1 Foreword

Few fields in cancer treatment have evolved so rapidly as breast cancer from a single, standardized treatment modality, as was mastectomy, to an extremely complex set of management steps in which surgery, radiotherapy, chemotherapy and hormonal therapy are intimately interlinked in their importance. The disease itself also covers tumors with very different biological behavior. This has made it absolutely necessary to standardize as much as possible the assessment of patient-related factors, the tumor characteristics, the treatment aspects and the factors used to evaluate outcome of therapy, as well concerning tumor control as side effects. Indeed, heterogeneity in the use of definitions, in any of these aspects could render the outcome of all studies useless and lead to the loss of important information as to statistically small, but clinically important effects.

This need has been perceived first of all in the clinical cooperative groups where specific questions are studied as to their prognostic importance and their therapeutic value. This has been the motivation to try to make an inventory of these elements in a "Manual for Breast Cancer Treatment". The first attempt has required a very big effort from the Breast Cancer Cooperative Group of the EORTC. The editions should certainly not be considered final but as outlines on which, with time, additions will be needed. The manual is giving a base from which further work will be easier. Certainly, at the rate the biological insight in the disease is evolving at present, it can be expected that it will be a continuously developing document and it is hoped that it will offer, in the future, a practical "state-of-the-art" presentation.

With its guidelines and its indications for systematic approach it will also be helpful to all clinicians, involved in the treatment of breast cancer. In this way, the clinical research which can only be carried out in a limited number of cancer centers, will support the development of a rigorous approach of the treatment of breast cancer in all hospitals and it can be hoped that this will be beneficial for all patients in Europe.

We apologize for errors and omissions, which will inevitably be present in this text and do ask suggestions for improvements which you might formulate when using this.

Emmanuel van der Schueren
Chairman Breast Cancer Cooperative Group at the time of the first edition, 1991

In the second (CD-ROM) edition some, streamlining rearrangements were made and some details were updated with the help of many of the former contributors. A chapter on hereditary breast cancer was added. A third (printed and CD-ROM) edition will be prepared to be distributed at the occasion of the next EORTC breast cancer working conference in Florence in 1998.

J.A. van Dongen, 1996

With the publication of this third (second CD-ROM and second printed) edition, presented at the first European Breast Cancer Conference, Florence 1998, we once again want to underline that correct assessment of all patient-, tumor- and therapy-related factors is crucial in breast cancer research.

Many of these items are still far from standardized through the different European study groups. Only use of common language and of same definitions will make information comparable and exchangable. From the commencement of EORTC activities the organization has promoted the principle of standardization of definitions; stimulated by the late Professor van der Shueren, the "manual" of the Breast Cancer Cooperative Group was written and the first edition published on the occasion of the fifth EORTC Breast Cancer Working Conference, Leuven 1991.

In this handbook we tried to describe carefully the meaning of words and principles used in breast cancer research and treatment.

We hope that this new edition of the manual will be helpful in reaching the goals formulated in 1991.

Since definitions should not change over time, much of the contents remain unchanged, but where necessary details were corrected; some rearrangements were thought useful and some paragraphs were added.

I want to thank the many colleagues who were helpful in preparing this edition, Excerpta Medica for their great activities in realizing the project and Pharmacia and Upjohn for the financial support.

J.A. van Dongen, 1998

The EORTC-Manual has gained credibility as a valuable source in research and management of breast cancer. The 4th edition (3rd Manual-in-Print and 3rd CD-ROM) is launched at the 2nd European Breast Cancer Conference, Brussels, 26–30 September 2000. The new edition of the Manual is a still growing collaboration between the EORTC Breast Cancer Cooperative Group and the EUSOMA (European Society of Mastology). A chapter on the sentinel node technique and criteria, the EUSOMA Florence Statement of 1998, and the 10 goals of Europa Donna have expanded the 4th edition. Several chapters have been revised radically in order to update information and to implement new management policies.

Further, in the CD-ROM, the chapter on Metastatic Disease is supported by guidelines for EORTC protocols on objective tumour response measured according to RECIST criteria. Moreover, the CD-ROM contains EUSOMA papers on future standards and minimum requirements regarding the set up of a Breast Unit, quality assurance in diagnostic assessment of breast diseases, and surgical options in the management of breast cancer.

The contributors to the Manual are all highly renowned European colleagues within the breast cancer research field. The author panel quite naturally undergoes alterations and new contributors have embarked on the list as seen from the acknowledgement inventory. It has been a great honour and privilege to serve and edit the EORTC Manual together with such a team of excellence. Finally, I would like to extend my gratitude to Excerpta Medica for their exceedingly professional help in making the Manual a worthy contribution to the field of breast cancer research and management.

Mogens Blichert-Toft, 2000

The treatment of a breast cancer becomes increasingly complex. The purpose of this manual as wished by professor van der Schueren in the first edition is to give a practical "state-of-the-art" presentation and to develop a common language and definitions which are needed for clinical research and to avoid misinterpretation by clinicians involved in the treatment of breast cancer. The slow but steady improvements in the treatment and research in breast cancer made this new edition necessary. Some chapters have been completely rewritten, among them, imaging, prognostic and predictive factors and adjuvant treatment. Furthermore, the Brussels and Barcelona statements have been added, following the consensus meetings of the second and third European Breast Cancer Conferences. These statements reflect the preoccupations of the scientific community. In Florence and Brussels, optimism was present: "Forging the way ahead for more research and better care in breast cancer", development of multidisciplinary breast clinics, screening, quality insurance, translational research and the eminent role of clinical trials.

In Barcelona, the tone has changed: "The future of breast cancer research in danger" expresses the fear of the participants that the necessary protection of the patient may in the future hamper the clinical and translational research by misevaluation of inexpert ethical committees and bureaucratic hurdles. The European directive planned to be active for May 2004 may even aggravate this situation. In the name of the EORTC breast cancer group, I want to thank my colleagues and friends who contributed to the update or rewrite of the chapters of this manual and also Emiel Rutgers, Jacek Jassem, Jolanda Remmelzwaal and Greenwich Medical Media for their editorial support. Further, Astra-Zeneca for their unrestricted educational grant that made the publication of this issue possible.

It has been a great honor to coordinate this fifth edition and to write the introduction that might be also the conclusion of my long EORTC activities!

Jean Pierre Julien, 2003

I.2 Florence statement – Forging the way ahead for more research on and better care in breast cancer

Introduction

The first European consensus on key issues in breast cancer has on Saturday 3 October 1998 been reached by nearly 1,000 clinicians, scientists and healthcare consumers attending a mass voting session at the 1st European Breast Cancer Conference (EBCC-1) in Florence. The Florence Statement sets the agenda for everyone involved in these key issues in breast cancer research, treatment, prevention and advocacy including the three major groups and organisers of EBCC-1:

–   The Breast Cancer Cooperative Group of the European Organization for the Research and Treatment of Cancer (EORTC-BCCG)
–   The European Society of Mastology (EUSOMA)
–   Europa Donna, the European Breast Cancer Coalition

This objective-setting document will stimulate much needed change in the field of breast cancer. EORTC-BCCG, EUSOMA and the patient-advocacy activities of Europa Donna will work towards these goals by lobbying European governments and mobilizing health-service providers, the scientific community and the healthcare industry. These new actions demanded by the EBCC-1 delegates will be assessed and reviewed in two years at EBCC-2, to be held in Brussels from 26 to 30 September, 2000.

Breast cancer is the commonest cancer and the most frequent cause of cancer death in women in every European Union country. Because of its importance and its potentially high curability, breast cancer deserves special attention and effort. The 1st European Breast Cancer Conference calls on the European Parliament to devote a plenary session to breast cancer. The Florence conference also makes the following statements:

On research:
–   Clinical trials are the mainstay for the development of optimal treatment of breast cancer and this conference is committed to encouraging maximum participation in clinical trials. Consumers should be fully involved at all stages in the design and conduct of clinical trials, by clear public information, discussion with ethics committees and increased accessibility to clinical trials.
–   This conference is committed to the application of pressure on governments, medical charities and the healthcare industry to invest more in breast cancer research, especially into translational studies. In addition, the major European charities are invited to co-ordinate their efforts to avoid unnecessary duplication of research programmes in different countries and thereby release resources to underpin European studies.

On genetic predisposition:
–   Given that knowledge about inherited predisposition to breast cancer is constantly emerging and that management options for mutation carriers are still not proven to be of benefit, the conference resolves that genetic testing should be undertaken in the setting of clinical research only. Such a setting needs personnel and facilities to study further the psychological effects and clinical outcomes in those who present for testing.
–   Genetic testing represents a potential threat to the privacy and security of women and could lead to commercial exploitation through gene patenting. The conference therefore demands national legislation and a European directive to protect women from personal, professional, financial or other discrimination.

On psychosocial status:
- This conference believes that the measurement of psychosocial status should be mandatory in the assessment and management of women's health and should not just be part of a clinical trial.

On treatment:
- This conference demands that those responsible for organising and funding breast cancer care ensure that all women have access to fully equipped multidisciplinary and multiprofessional breast clinics based on populations of around 250,000.

On quality of care:
- Given the importance of the quality of surgery, radiotherapy and chemotherapy in determining outcome, quality-assurance programmes should become mandatory for breast cancer services to qualify for funding from healthcare providers.
- Evidence-based multidisciplinary management guidelines defined at national and European level with the consensus of healthcare professionals, voluntary organizations, other health-service providers and consumers will further improve outcome.

Professor **Luigi Cataliotti**   Professor **Cornelis van de Velde**   Mrs **Gloria Freilich**
President EUSOMA   Chairman EORTC-BCCG   President Europa Donna

I.3   Brussels statement

Introduction

The second European Breast cancer conference reached a consensus on several key issues during the closing plenary session on the 30th September 2000 in Brussels. Clinicians, scientists, and healthcare consumers representing 3150 participants used a computerised voting system in plenary session to formulate the *Brussels Statement.*

This document sets the agenda for the future activities of the three major groups involved in breast cancer research, treatment, prevention and advocacy:

–   The Breast Cancer Group of the European Organization for Research and Treatment in Cancer (EORTC-BCG)
–   The European Society of Mastology (EUSOMA)
–   Europa Donna, the European Breast Cancer Coalition

It is hoped that the objectives outlined in this document will stimulate much-needed change in the field of breast cancer. EORTC-BCG, EUSOMA together with the breast cancer advocacy activities of EUROPA DONNA, will work towards these goals by lobbying European Governments and the European Commission and by mobilising health-service providers, the scientific community and the health-care industry. These measures called for by EBCC-2 delegates will be assessed and reviewed at EBCC-3 to be held in Barcelona in March 2002.

Breast cancer is the commonest cancer and the most frequent cause of cancer death in women throughout Europe. Because of its importance and its potential for successful treatment, breast cancer deserves special attention and effort. The Brussels conference makes the following statements:

Breast cancer should be managed in multidisciplinary clinics

Following the Florence Statement that established that all women should have access to fully equipped, dedicated breast units, the three Societies have produced European Guidelines defining the requirements for such units. These European guidelines stress the importance of multidisciplinarity (ie the collaboration between surgeons, radiologists, clinicians, pathologists, etc.) and multiprofessionality (ie the collaboration between doctors, nurses, psychologists, social workers, etc.).

The Conference demands that national governments establish and accredit breast units in their countries in accordance with the Guidelines and ensure that breast cancer diagnosis and care are carried out in those units.

All breast units should develop quality assurance programmes entering their data onto a common European database. The Conference pleads for all the breast units to collect data on incidence and mortality and to pool them in a common European database.

Breast cancer screening

The conference acknowledges the important contribution made by mammographic screening to decreasing mortality and improving breast cancer care. All women should be offered full information about the benefits and risks of mammographic screening.

All European women between the age of 50 and 75 should be offered quality-assured *mammographic* breast screening free at the point of delivery. Programmes should not be provided without adequate provision for assessment and treatment of screen-detected abnormalities.

Quality assurance in breast cancer research

The Conference wishes to stress the importance of quality assurance procedures as an integral part of the conduct of studies for all involved disciplines. It invites health service providers and research funding agencies to consider the additional cost for quality assurance procedures as an investment to obtain better outcomes.

Researchers and clinical investigators should recognise the ethical and scientific necessity of always including quality assurance procedures in their study protocols.

Risk assessment

The Conference wishes to bring to everyone's attention the increasing potentials offered by new methods to assess breast cancer risk for an individual woman and encourages researchers to identify a standardised risk-assessment methodology suitable for European women. This will facilitate research in preventive measures such as mammography and innovative imaging modalities, lifestyle modifications, chemoprevention, and prophylactic surgery.

In addressing the issue of genetic testing the Conference agreed that not all women with a family history are at high risk and necessarily need or want a genetic test.

Genetic testing should be provided only after receiving appropriate specialist counselling. The Conference expresses the opinion that genetic testing should not be encouraged in the absence of protective legislation against socio-economic discrimination.

Treatment tailoring

The Conference welcomes the progress made in tailoring treatment programmes to individual patients and acknowledges the fact that a great contribution to this progress comes from translational research (i.e. those studies which result from the interaction between laboratory and clinical research).

The Conference wishes to assist in the coming years to a great development of translational research in breast cancer by means of well-funded research projects on frozen tumour specimens for which free circulation among different countries should also be ensured. Legislators on data protection are asked to facilitate this scientific evolution by recognising the importance of these studies.

Informed consented collection of frozen tumour specimens should be obtained from all breast cancer patients as a routine procedure.

Participation in clinical trials

Randomized clinical trials represent the most effective way of evaluating new therapies but also offer optimal treatment opportunities. Positive steps should be taken to minimise obstacles to the participation both for patients and clinicians.

Press, broadcasting media and internet providers are invited to increase awareness of the importance of participation in clinical trials as the most important contribution to the progress of medicine and the best option for maximum quality care.

Health authorities and research agencies should give adequate support to national and international data centres conducting clinical trials in breast cancer.

Martine Piccart
Conference Chair

Gloria Freilich
Conference Co-Chair

Luigi Cataliotti
President EUSOMA

Mary Buchanan
President Europa Donna

Jacek Jassem
President EORTC-Breast Group

I.4   Barcelona Statement – The future of breast cancer research in danger

Introduction

This statement has been prepared by the scientific committee of the 3rd European breast cancer conference that was held in Barcelona from the 19th the 23rd March 2002. This follows an open debate by the participants of the conference at a plenary session on Saturday the 23rd March. The agenda for this discussion had been set by the scientific committee following private discussions where we recognised that there was a pan-European concern about the future of clinical and translational research for cancer in general and breast cancer in particular.

Breast cancer in Europe

Breast cancer is the commonest malignancy amongst women in Europe and the commonest cause of death amongst women in their middle years, although in some parts of Europe, with increasing tobacco consumption carcinoma of the lung is beginning to catch up or even overtake breast cancer as a cause of premature death.

Currently there are 321,000 new cases of breast cancer diagnosed in Europe each year and this is associated with 124,000 deaths. The trends in age specific mortality across Europe demonstrate remarkable patterns [1]. These were discussed in detail at a special session set aside to consider the matter. The data were presented by Professor Sir Richard Peto, following which there were three separate talks attempting to explain the trends in mortality according to socio-economic and lifestyle changes, the stage of diagnosis and improvements in treatment.

Across most of Europe there has been a steep increase in age specific mortality from breast cancer from the early post-war years until the mid 1980's. This almost certainly can be accounted for by increasing prosperity as the steepness of the rise was determined by the baseline socio-economic deprivation in the late 1940's and early 1950's. In addition lifestyle changes whereby professional women have been postponing the age of first pregnancy could also account for some of the rise in incidence and mortality from the 1960's onwards. Mortality rates started to plateau in the mid 1980's and in many countries throughout Europe there has been a significant fall in age specific mortality between 1987 and the year 2000. The steepest fall, amounting to approximately 30% has been witnessed in the UK [2].

Explanations for this fall in mortality are complex. It is difficult, if not impossible to explain any of this fall to socio-economic or lifestyle trends. Some could be attributed to early diagnosis as a result of the screening programmes which began to be introduced in the late 80's early 90's but they would not be expected to deliver their full potential before the late 90's. Nevertheless the breast cancer awareness programmes linked to mammographic screening may have encouraged many women to present with their disease at a clinically less advanced stage.

That aside there was a consensus that something like two thirds in breast cancer mortality since the late 1980's can be attributed to improvements in treatment. It can be no coincidence that the first world overview of adjuvant systemic therapy was presented to the scientific community in 1985 [3] and treatments such as tamoxifen for post-menopausal women and cytotoxic chemotherapy for pre-menopausal women were rapidly introduced at

that stage, which explains why the fall in mortality has been witnessed across all age groups, not just the post-menopausal women who are involved in the screening programmes.

Following the 1985 world overview there have been an increasing number of multi-centre randomised controlled trials for the treatment of early breast cancer involving collaborative groups throughout Europe with results that continue to demonstrate modest but incremental improvements. If implemented these newer modalities of therapy should contribute to a continuing downward trend in mortality throughout Europe.

There are many exciting new agents and therapeutic strategies that are awaiting formal evaluation by means of the randomised controlled trial. Yet this very mechanism, which has proven the benefits of treatment in the past and contributed to at least two thirds of the fall in mortality over the last fifteen years, is under threat by well meaning but misguided bureaucratic challenges.

The protection of the individual patient from abuse is the first priority

There has been a long and tragic history of the abuse of human subjects in the name of medical science. This dates back to the Nazi war criminals and the Nuremberg trials. That so-called medical research was nothing other than torture and the "science" was so seriously flawed that even out of all this human suffering, nothing of worth can be retrieved [4]. To make sure that these tragedies will never happen again we have had a number of ethical guidelines pre-eminent amongst which is the Declaration of Helsinki of the World Health Organisation.

Added to that we must not forget the thalidomide tragedy, resulting from the inadequate testing of a drug with appalling consequences to new-born babies. Then again it is essential to protect patient's confidentiality, which might be at risk by the exchange of notes and clinical details necessary for the conduct of clinical trials and finally there have been some well-publicised examples of scientific fraud, misleading the public and causing untold harm. The most high profile of these was the fraudulent trial of high dose chemotherapy in South Africa [5].

These unquestioned abuses of human subjects have to be defended against but there is always the danger that the entirely appropriate and well meaning structures, guidelines and ethical directives might have unintentional consequences in the future.

It is our concern that the over-reaction to abuses in the past has erected so many bureaucratic hurdles as to make the future conduct of legitimate clinical research exceedingly difficult or prohibitively expensive.

Obstacles to progress

Perhaps the most obvious obstacle to progress for randomised controlled trials in the treatment of breast cancer is the process known as good clinical practice (GCP). Even the term GCP is sinister in the way it has hijacked the meaning of words to suit the bureaucratic needs. There is nothing about the process of "good clinical practice" that can be taken as guidelines for the practice of good clinical medicine. In other words GCP has Orwellian overtones suggestive of 1984 where the very meaning of words has been distorted as to make rational thinking impossible.

Its intention is to protect patient confidentiality, ensure that all the ethical imperatives have been adhered to and guarantee that no rare but important adverse side effects of a new therapy will be overlooked. No one can argue against these lofty ideals, but the reality in practice is making the conduct of clinical trials according to GCP principles very difficult for the academic community and prohibitively expensive unless interpreted liberally. We would therefore urge the regulatory authorities to constantly revisit these issues and accept that the process is far from perfect at present. No one would wish the "law of unintended consequences" to apply, so that the very control mechanisms to police clinical research end up in extinguishing the flame of progress.

Ethical control

No one would dispute that good ethics and good science must go hand in hand. The original declaration of Helsinki was noble in its intent but subsequent versions have tightened controls and made the informed consent procedures so threatening both to the patient and the scientist as to discourage recruitment of the large numbers of patients which are required for statistical confidence. No one would deny the ethical principle of autonomy and the right to self-determination but societies cannot expect to give individuals their rights without in return the individual shouldering their responsibilities.

It could be argued therefore that if patients in the future demand better treatments than those in the past there is a moral responsibility to act as equal partners with the clinical scientists in the quest for the cure for cancer. There is a price to pay for autonomy but it ignores responsibility and this can be calculated in terms of unnecessary loss of life from cancer in the future [6].

The Ethics Committees themselves that have to interpret and administer the declaration and codes of conduct governing clinical research cannot be populated by individuals who are mere tokens. The study of medical ethics is a scholarly subject. It is not intuitive and those who are granted the privilege of serving on these committees also have the responsibility to acquaint themselves with the nature of disease, the principles of the scientific method and an understanding of the philosophical underpinning of medical ethics.

If these Ethics Committees (institutional review bodies) do not accept their responsibility to encourage the future of cancer research they can be perceived as obstacles to progress, carrying equal responsibility for unnecessary loss of life in the future, as those clinical scientists who have abused the trust of the public in the past.

Translational research

As we are entering the era of "molecular medicine", it becomes a high priority to understand why some patients benefit from the therapies and some don't.

We now have in our hands new and very powerful tools, such as genomics and proteomics that should greatly facilitate this task and lead to greatly improved treatment individualisation in a not too distant future.

But this dream will never become a reality if translational research is not "facilitated": in other words, individual tumor profiles must be obtained in the context of clinical trials, analysed in the laboratory and correlated to clinical outcome.

The creation of this essential "link" between clinicians and laboratory scientists can only happen if (A) patients understand its importance for the advancement of patient-care, (B) physicians are encouraged – and not discouraged – to devote extra time and efforts in this direction and (C) governments give financial support to these initiatives, which will not always be viewed as serving the interests of the Pharmaceutical Industry and, therefore, are better financed through an independent channel.

A very constructive proposal from Europa Donna representatives and deserving to be examined in more detail is the suggestion to incorporate consent for any sound translational research, whether carried out today or several years from now, in the clinical trial consent form, as long as it does not involve germline mutation studies.

The practical implication for this would be a simplified consent procedure, while the very few patients not willing to have their tumours analysed would be allowed to express this disagreement in a written document.

The way ahead

One of the most heartening aspects of the European Breast Cancer Conferences starting with the first in Florence and culminating in the third in Barcelona has been the emergence of Europa Donna, the European Breast Cancer Coalition as a force to be reckoned with. Led by their President, Dr Mary Buchanan, and Vice President, Stella Kyriakides, their representatives have demonstrated a willingness and enthusiasm to be advocates for clinical trials as well as advocates for the needs of individual patients. In return for their support they make the legitimate plea that the patients themselves should be seen as equal partners and stakeholders in the fight against breast cancer.

We have now reached a very important crossroad in the history of clinical research for breast cancer, which will no doubt be reflected across the whole spectrum of malignant disease in the not too distant future. The sufferers themselves recognise that it is in their enlightened self-interest to take part in clinical trials because patients treated within clinical trials tend to do better than those treated outside [7]. In addition the Europa Donna advocates recognise that as they are beneficiaries of volunteers for clinical trials in the past, they should contribute to the advance of knowledge for the next generation, many of whom might be their own daughters.

It is therefore essential to build on the vision that emerged from the Barcelona Conference, to set up networks and partnership groups where the consumer could be involved in the design and the monitoring of the clinical trial as well as being passive subjects within the clinical trial. EUROPA DONNA is already advancing well along these lines and has gained further encouragement from the cooperation and enhanced acceptance at EBCC-3.

To achieve this requires an education programme targeted at laywomen, concerning the nature of science and the nature of malignant disease. Such an educational programme must target the young as well as the middle aged.

A similar education programme must also be targeted on future members of ethics committees and institutional review bodies who will sit in judgment of the clinical scientists in the future. Last but not least the politicians who are directly or indirectly responsible for the bureaucracy governing drug development and drug registration must be taught to have a longer vision than the instant popularity they seek in anticipation of the next election. For a start those responsible for "good clinical practice" must revisit this hydra headed monster in order to determine how it can be trimmed down in order to facilitate clinical research, rather than impeding it. We believe that this can be achieved with absolutely no threat to the patient providing common sense is allowed to prevail.

Conclusion

In conclusion this declaration of Barcelona, once more commits the clinical scientific community within Europe to progress in the search for the cure for breast cancer. At every step on the way this quest must ensure the protection of the individual patient and guarantee that her needs are pre-eminent above and beyond the needs of the clinical trial itself. Yet at the same time we believe that it is in the enlightened self- interest of the individual patients to be associated with the clinical trial process and this is now recognised by the women's advocacy groups themselves.

The way forward therefore is to build on the strengths of the past where Europe has led the world in the discovery of better treatments for carcinoma of the breast. At the same time we must recognize the dangers and obstacles to progress in the future. Many of these obstacles are self-imposed and are the unintentional consequences of processes introduced to protect the patient from the abuses that were prevalent in the past.

To achieve this, education has to be the watchword and that is education of the lay public and the ethics committees as well as education of the next generation of clinical scientists.

The next watchword is partnership and this partnership must be more than lip service to an ideal but a genuine mutual respect between the clinical scientist, their patients and the politicians responsible for the bureaucracy governing the discovery and registration of new therapies. GCP like tax and death is inevitable in one form or another but this must not be perceived, as an obstacle to progress and the funding for GCP should not make the cost of the clinical trial prohibitive. If necessary it should be funded through tax revenue from central government rather than being seen as a burden upon the clinical academic establishment and the cancer charities.

Perhaps part of the solution to many of these problems is contained within the words of Stella Kyriakides from her Europa Donna plenary lecture on Friday the 22nd March:

> "Life with Breast Cancer has slowly acquired a new meaning- it is slowly being associated with having a voice, with learning to raise it effectively by asking the correct questions,by demanding to be given valid and informative answers, by working hand in hand with all involved, by having hope in new treatments,by remaining realistic about the seriousness of the disease,by not forgetting those who lose their lives to it, by looking into the future with hope.
>
> There is no longer 'a feeling of despair created by the imagination which pretends there is a future' as Dubois once said, there actually IS a future. A future that allows us to enjoy every moment at hand, that allows planning for millions of moments and thousands of days ahead.
>
> I really am not sure that we are survivors – some of us are patients, some have had the experience – of one thing I am sure, all of us here today, in this Odyssey, must be and are, PARTNERS. PARTNERSHIP IS WHAT IS ACTUALLY EMBODIED IN THE ORGANISA-TION OF THIS CONFERENCE BY EORTC,EUSOMA and EUROPA DONNA.
>
> So let us all work hand in hand, as partners, to make life with breast cancer acquire its real meaning, achieve its true potential and create a future for every person faced with this reality."

Michael Baum
Conference Chair

José Baselga
Conference Co-Chair

Luigi Cataliotti
President, EUSOMA

Mary Buchanan
President, Europa Donna

Jacek Jassem
President, EORTC BCG

Martine Piccart
Past Conference Chair

References

1. Bray F, Sankila R, Ferlay J, Parkin DM. "Estimates of cancer incidence and mortality in Europe in 1995", EJC 38 (2002), 1; 99–166
2. Peto, R., Boreham, J., Clarke M., et al. UK and USA breast cancer deaths down 25% in year 2000 at ages 29–60 years. *Lancet* 2000; 355: 1822
3. Early Breast Cancer Trialists' Collaborative Group. Effects of adjuvant tamoxifen and of cytotoxic therapy on mortality in early breast cancer. An overview of 61 randomized trials among 28,896 women. *N Engl J Med* 1988; 319: 1681–1692
4. Hanauske-Abel HM. Not a slippery slope or sudden subversion: German Medicine and National Socialism in 1933. *Brit Med J* 1996;313: 1453–63
5. Weiss, R., Rifkin, R.M., Stewart F.M., et al. High-dose chemotherapy for high-risk primary breast cancer: an on-site review of the Bezwoda study *The Lancet* 2000; 355: 999–1003
6. Baum, M., and Vaidya, J., The price of autonomy. Health Expectations, 1999; 2: 78–81
7. BMA, Patients taking part in clinical trials do better. http://www.bma.org.uk/ap.nsf June 2002

II. General assessment

II.1 Performance status

II.2 Menstrual status

II.3 Age categories in breast cancer studies

II.4 Date and definition of primary diagnosis

II.1 Performance status

a. The *WHO performance status scale (ECOG scale)* is used as a reference:

   0 Able to carry out all normal activity without restriction.
   1 Restricted in physically strenuous activity but ambulatory and able to carry out light work.
   2 Ambulatory and capable of all self-care activity but unable to carry out any work, up and about more than 50% of waking hours.
   3 Capable of only limited self-care, confined to bed or chair more than 50% of waking hours.
   4 Completely disabled, cannot carry on any self-care, totally confined to bed or chair.

b. Frequently the *Karnofsky scale* is used:

Description	Scale (%)
Normal, no complaint	100
Able to carry on normal activities; minor signs or symptoms of disease	90
Normal activity with effort	80
Capable of self-care. Unable to carry on normal activity or to do active work	70
Ambulatory. Requires some assistance but able to care for most of own needs	60
Requires considerable assistance and frequent medical care	50
Disabled. Requires special care and assistance	40
Severely disabled. Hospitalization indicated though death is not imminent	30
Very sick. Hospitalization necessary. Active supportive treatment necessary	20
Moribund	10
Dead	0

II.2 Menstrual status

Unless the protocol requires menstrual status to be more specifically determined, patients are considered to be postmenopausal in the following situations:

– amenorrhea for longer than 12 months irrespective of age; or
– amenorrhea for longer than six months and age older than or equal to 50 years; or
– bilateral oophorectomy irrespective of age; or
– radiation castration with amenorrhea for longer than three months irrespective of age; or
– hysterectomy and age older than or equal to 55 years; or
– patients using HRT or oral contraceptives and age older than or equal to 55 years.

For patients hysterectomized or using HRT/oral contraceptives and aged below 55 years, menstrual status should be determined by measurement of FSH and LH performed at least four weeks after stopping HRT/oral contraceptives. The reference definition should be according to the postmenopausal range of the individual laboratories.

II.3 Age categories in breast cancer studies

a. Background

The biology of breast cancer is different in different age groups. This necessitates in many studies stratification for age categories; for some research questions, different study design is necessary for specific age groups.

Breast cancer is a slowly growing tumor. The number of available years at risk is important when studies are designed; this is especially crucial in primary treatment studies, in particular in studies for (very) early disease (e.g. DCIS) and might be reason to exclude elderly patients (over 75 years) for such protocols.

Comorbidity and risk for serious side effects from chemotherapy is increasing with (old) age. This is an argument to exclude elderly patients from many chemotherapy trials and to design special studies for chemotherapy in the elderly.

Sensitivity for hormonal treatment and possibly tumor growth rate are influenced by the hormonal status. Hence, differentiation between pre- and postmenopausal categories is logical. For practical reasons this is in some studies translated into age of below or over 50 years but for EORTC studies, menstrual status should be defined according to II.2 guidelines.

Some suggested that young age may be related with poor prognosis. Many studies hint to an age effect on breast cancer recurrence risk (high in the very young patients) after breast-conserving therapy. Using age separation seems to be mandatory for breast con-servation studies.

b. Age cut-off levels to be used in breast cancer protocols

Young/others	35 years
Premenopausal/postmenopausal	50 years (EORTC: see II.2)
Elderly/others	75 years
Exclusion in "aggressive" chemotherapy trials	Over 60 years

II.4 Date and definition of primary diagnosis

The date of diagnosis is the date of the tissue biopsy on which the diagnosis of breast cancer is confirmed for the first time. This can be either a tru-cut needle biopsy or any form of incisional or excisional biopsy.

If only a fine needle aspiration has been performed or a fine needle aspiration preceded a positive biopsy, the date of the first fine needle aspiration at which grade V cytology is observed is the date of diagnosis. In the absence of tissue for histology, the result of cytology should be in accordance with clinical and mammographic findings. In cases where histologic and/or cytologic confirmation of the diagnosis of breast cancer is missing, the patient cannot be included in breast cancer studies.

III. Breast cancer screening

III.1 Screening options

With the high incidence of breast cancer and mammography being an "easy" diagnostic tool with high sensitivity and specificity, population-based breast cancer screening is in many countries considered to be cost-effective for age category 50–75.

Offered (imposed) screening has special ethical aspects and creates maximal responsibility for optimal treatment. The women recruited for screening and the patients discovered by screening are selected groups. This selection has impact on the screening research and on treatment research.

a. Nation-wide screening programs
All women – of certain age category – are invited on a regular basis for screening.

b. Local screening programs
Women of a certain region or city are invited.

c. Open – walk-in – screening centers
Facility for breast cancer screening. Recruitment of clients by advertisement.

III.2   Studies to evaluate screening

a.   End points

- decrease of breast cancer mortality in screened population
- decrease of T stage and N stage in the comparison of screened and unscreened populations
- increase of *in situ* lesions in this comparison

b.   Options to study effectiveness of screening

- randomization of individuals to be invited
- randomization of groups/countries/cities to be invited
- comparing outcome with like populations or with historical data
- breast cancer mortality trend in population

c.   Main points to be studied when evaluating screening programs

- age category and interval between screening rounds
- compliance (per age group)
- referral rate
- biopsy rate
- overall cancer detection rate
- stage of detected cancers
- positive predictive value of test
- positive predictive value of biopsy
- interval cancers
- details of used technique (type and number of views [in first and in following rounds], way of invitation, single- or double-reading etc.)
- quality control systems
- use apart from mammography of physical examination and/or of questionnaires
- use of special breast clinics for further work-up and treatment
- calculation of costs

d.   Basic items having impact on screening benefit

- lead time bias: diagnosis earlier than in clinical cancer; impact on survival measurement
- length bias: slow growing tumors are picked up better than fast growing tumors; impact also because of possible differences in tumor biology, depending the growth rate
- self-selection bias: special subpopulations may have better compliance; due to their risk situation and e.g. life expectancy impact on possible benefit
- the increasing use of mammography in general and the *a priori* follow-up situation of some risk groups may detract from the benefit of population-based screening.

Reference

www.euref.org

IV.   Assessment before primary treatment

IV.1   Classification of tumour, regional nodes and metastases: staging

IV.2   Minimal requirements to exclude distant metastases

IV.3   Standardisation of the diagnostic evaluation of the breast

IV.4   Prognostic and predictive factors

IV.1 Classification of tumour, regional nodes and metastases: staging

Introduction

– Clinical measurement and classification of primary breast cancer is done since 1958 according to the UICC/TNM classification. The original classification was modified several times. Sixth edition [1a] was published in 2002 and the new classification should be used since January 2003 (ongoing trials should employ the classification used when the trial was activated).

   In publications, the used TNM system should be mentioned explicitly. The pTNM classification adds to the accuracy of the classification of the breast cancer. This classification is more complex and evolving with the development of imaging techniques, the sentinel node dissection and the increased use of immunohistochemical and molecular techniques.

– Every breast cancer should be confirmed by the triple diagnosis: clinical assessment, result of mammography and result of cytology or preferably histologically (tru-cut, open biopsy) and consistent with the imaging results.

– Classification is the same for female and male breast cancer.

– In case of multiple simultaneous primary tumours in one breast, the tumour with the highest T category should be used for classification.

– Simultaneous bilateral breast cancers should be classified independently.

– The anatomical sub-site of origin should be recorded but not considered in classification.

a. Anatomical sub sites

Breast

– In the UICC-TNM classification the localisation of a tumour is indicated by using numbers:

   0 = Nipple
   1 = Central portion
   2 = Upper inner quadrant
   3 = Lower-inner quadrant
   4 = Upper-outer quadrant
   5 = Lower-outer quadrant
   6 = Axillary tail

Central tumours are those situated or partly situated in the retroareolar zone. Axillary tail is the part of the breast outside the circle limiting the four quadrants. When the lesion extends over two quadrants, the quadrant containing the main part of the tumour is identified.

If the definition of the localisation is considered critical, and to keep the UICC/TMN numbers, the EORTC Breast Cancer Group suggest to add a second definition for a tumour located in two regions.

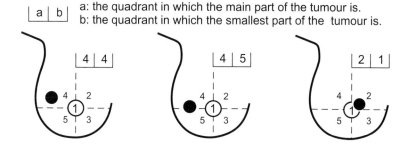

a | b   a: the quadrant in which the main part of the tumour is.
         b: the quadrant in which the smallest part of the tumour is.

For a lesion over two quadrants but also retroareolar, only retroareolar lesion and the quadrant with the main part of the tumour should be coded.

Paget disease should be coded $\boxed{0 \quad 0}$, or if associated with a central lesion on the mammogram $\boxed{0 \quad 1}$.

Nodes

1. Axillary – The axilla can be divided into the following levels:
   - Level 1 (low axilla). Lymph nodes lateral to the lateral border of pectoralis minor muscle
   - Level 2 (mid axilla). Lymph nodes between the medial and lateral border of the pectoralis minor muscle. This level includes the interpectoral (Rotter) nodes.
   - Level 3 (apical axilla). Lymph nodes medial to the medial margin of pectoralis minor muscle.

   These "standard" levels of axillary specimens can only be indicated by the operator and are difficult to distinguish in the "en bloc" specimen of the axilla unless special marks are used. Therefore, this procedure should be strongly recommended. Intramammary lymph nodes are coded as axillary lymph nodes.
2. Infraclavicular (subclavicular) ipsilateral lymph nodes.
3. Internal mammary ipsilateral lymph nodes in the intercostals spaces along the edge of the sternum in the endothoracic facia.
4. Supraclavicular ipsilateral lymph nodes.
   - Any other lymph node metastasis is coded as distant metastasis (M1), including cervical or controlateral internal mammary lymph nodes.

b.   UICC/TNM system

TNM clinical classification
T: Primary tumour
   - Tx: Primary tumour cannot be assessed.
   - T0:   No evidence of primary tumour.
   - Tis: Carcinoma in situ.
     - Tis (dcis): Ductal carcinoma in situ.
     - Tis (lcis): Lobular carcinoma in situ.
     - Tis (Paget): Paget disease of the nipple with no tumour.

T1:   Tumour 2 cm or less in greatest dimension.
   - T1 mic: microinvasion 0.1cm or less in greatest dimension.
   - T1a: more than 0.1 cm but not more than 0.5 cm in greatest dimension.
   - T1b: more than 0.5 cm but not more than 1 cm in greatest dimension.
   - T1c: more than 1 cm but not more than 2 cm in greatest dimension.

T2:   more than 2 cm but not more than 5 cm in greatest dimension.
T3:   more than 5 cm in greatest dimension.
T4:   Tumour of any size with direct extension to chest wall or skin only as described in T4a to T4d.
   - T4a: extension to chest wall.
   - T4b: oedema (including peau d'orange) or ulceration of the skin of the breast or satellite skin nodule confined to the same breast.
   - T4c: both 4a and 4b, as above.
   - T4d: inflammatory carcinoma.

N: Regional lymph nodes
- Nx: Regional lymph nodes cannot be assessed (e. g., previously removed).
- N0: No regional lymph nodes metastasis.
- N1: Metastasis in movable ipsilateral axillary lymph node(s).
- N2: Metastasis in fixed ipsilateral axillary lymph node(s) or in clinically apparent ipsilateral internal mammary lymph node(s) in the absence of clinically evident axillary lymph node metastasis.
- N3: Metastasis in ipsilateral infraclavicular lymph node(s) with or without axillary lymph node involvement or in clinically apparent ipsilateral internal mammary lymph node(s) in the presence of clinically evident axillary lymph node metastasis; or metastasis in ipsilateral supraclavicular lymph node(s) with or without axillary or internal mammary lymph nodes involvement.
    - N3a: metastasis in infraclavicular lymph node(s).
    - N3b: metastasis in internal mammary and axillary lymph nodes.
    - N3c: metastasis in supraclavicular lymph nodes.

M: Distant metastasis
- Mx: distant metastasis cannot be assessed.
- M0: no distant metastasis.
- M1: distant metastasis.

pTNM pathological classification
pT categories correspond to the T categories.
pN:
- pNx: Regional lymph nodes cannot be assessed (not removed for study or previously removed)
- pN0: No regional lymph nodes metastasis.
- pN1mi: Micro metastasis (larger than 0.2 mm but none larger than 2 mm in greatest dimension)
- pN1: Metastasis in 1–3 ipsilateral axillary lymph node(s) and/or in ipsilateral internal mammary nodes with microscopic metastasis detected by sentinel lymph node but not clinically apparent.
    - pN1a: metastasis in 1–3 axillary lymph node(s) including at least one larger than 2 mm in greatest dimension
    - pN1b: internal mammary lymph nodes with microscopic metastasis detected by sentinel lymph nodes dissection but not clinically apparent.
    - pN1c: metastasis in 1–3 axillary lymph node(s) and internal mammary lymph nodes with microscopic metastasis detected by sentinel lymph nodes dissection but not clinically apparent.
- pN2: Metastasis in 4–9 ipsilateral axillary lymph nodes or in clinically apparent ipsilateral internal mammary lymph node(s) in the absence of axillary lymph nodes metastasis.
    - pN2a: Metastasis in 4–9 ipsilateral axillary lymph nodes includind at least one that is larger than 2 mm.
    - pN2b: Metastasis in clinically apparent internal mammary lymph node(s) in the absence of axillary lymph node metastasis.
- pN3: Metastasis in 10 or more ipsilateral axillary lymph nodes or in ipsisteral infraclavicular lymph nodes; or in clinically apparent ipsilateral internal mammary lymph nodes in the presence of one or more positive axillary lymph nodes; or in more than 3 axillary lymph nodes with clinically negative microscopic metastasis in internal mammary lymph nodes; or in ipsilateral supraclavicular lymph nodes.

- pN3a: metastasis in 10 or more axillary lymph nodes (at least one larger than 2 mm) or metastasis in infranclavicular lymph nodes.
- pN3b: metastasis in clinically apparent internal mammary lymph node(s) in the presence of positive axillary lymph node(s) ; or metastasis in more than 3 axillary lymph nodes and in internal mammary lymph nodes with microscopic metastasis detected by sentinel lymph node dissection but not clinically apparent.
- pN3c: metastasis in supraclavicular lymph node(s).

pM: categories correspond to the M categories.

Stage grouping

Stage 0	Tis	N0	M0
Stage 1	TI*	N0	M0
Stage IIA	T0	N1	M0
	T1*	N1	M0
	T2	N0	M0
Stage IIB	T2	N1	M0
	T3	N0	M0
Stage IIIA	T0	N2	M0
	T1*	N2	M0
	T2	N2	M0
	T3	N1, N2	M0
Stage IIIB	T4	N0, N1, N2	M0
Stage IIIC	Any T	N3	M0
Stage V	Any T	Any N	M1

Note: *T1 included T1mic.

c.   *Addendum to T primary tumour*

- Measurement of the tumour by calliper is imprecise and often inadequate as many tumour are now very small or detected only by mammography. A certainty factor (C factor) is available in the TNM classification. For breast cancer C1 corresponds to the evidence from mammography; C2: evidence from ultrasonography.
  T...C1: mammographic size, T... C2: ultrasonic size.
  The EORTC recommends to register the clinical size, mammographic size and if done, the ultrasonic measurement.
- The pT measure in the UICC/TNM classification is: "no gross tumour at the margins of resection". Microscopic measurement is advocated by the EORTC. The technique of measurement should be mentioned explicitly.
- Tis is a difficult item for clinical evaluation and in fact the designation of only pTis is an insufficient indicator for therapy planning. It is therefore mandatory also for in situ lesions to mention the mammographical and the pathological size.
- pT should relate only to the invasive component: an invasive lesion of less than 0.5 cm, even with an extended in situ component (EIC), will be a pT1a. The EORTC advise to estimate also the size of the tumour including EIC: maximal distance between edges of intraductal extensions.

- Tmic (in fact pTmic): microinvasion is the extension of tumour cells beyond the basement membrane into the adjacent tissues with no focus more than 0.1 cm in greatest dimension. When there are multiple foci of micro invasion do not use the sum of all individual foci but note the multifocality.
- T4a. Chest wall includes ribs, intercostal muscles and seratus anterior muscle but not pectoralis muscles.
- Inflammatory carcinoma. According to the UICC/TNM description, inflammatory carcinoma is characterized by diffuse brawny indurations of the skin with an erysipeloïd edge, usually with no underlying mass. For practical reasons, the EORTC uses the clinical definition of inflammatory breast cancer: redness over at least one third of the breast and a positive FNA aspiration or skin biopsy or tru-cut biopsy. Dimpling of the skin, simple retraction or other skin changes except those in T4 core and T4d may occur in T1, T2, T3 without affecting the classification.

e. Addendum to regional lymph nodes

- infraclavicular (subclavicular) = Level III (apex) and coded now: N3a
- N2b "clinically apparent": detected by clinical examination or by imaging studies excluding lymphoscintigraphy.
- The number of nodes examined should be registered
- When size is a criterium for pN classification, measurement of the metastasis and not of the entire lymph node should be made.
- The classification based solely on sentinel node biopsy without subsequent axillary dissection should be designated pN0(sn) or pN1(sn).
- Isolated tumour cells (ITC): single tumour cells or small clusters of cells <0.2 mm in greatest dimension with generally no evidence of metastatic activity (e.g. proliferation of stromal reaction). ITC detected by immunohistochemistry should be designated pN0(i−) or pN0(i+). ITC detected by molecular biology should be designated pN0(mol−) or pN0(mol+).

f. Addendum to stage grouping

- Locally advanced disease. The terminology of locally advanced disease is widely used without generally accepted definition or description. Breast cancer has become locally advanced as a result of growth pattern of primary tumour, lymph node metastasis or signs of inflammation. Tumour dependent factors:
  - Extension of the tumour to the chest wall: T4a
  - Oedema (including peau d'orange): T4b
  - Ulceration: T4b
  - Satellite skin nodules: T4b
  - Inflammatory: T4d; for specific criteria see paragraph d.

Regional node dependent factors:
Metastasis in lymph nodes: infraclavicular or internal mammary and axillary or supraclavicular: N3.

IV.2 Minimal requirements to exclude distant metastasis

In order to conclude that the patient is free of distant metastasis at primary diagnosis of breast cancer (M0), the following minimal requirements are demanded:

– Clinically detectable distant metastasis at primary diagnosis of stage I and II (Tis-1–2, N0-1) breast cancer is uncommon. Therefore, in the absence of signs and symptoms of distant metastasis found on history-taking or physical examination, no further diagnostic methods are required to exclude distant metastasis.

– In all higher stages of the primary tumour, the examination at primary diagnosis should consist of history and physical examination, complemented by chest X-ray, bone scintigraphy, alkaline phosphatase (AP) and gamma glutamyl transferase (gamma-GT). Other possible diagnostic tools (liver ultrasound, CT scan, bone radiograms, MRI, PET scan) should be used only when indicated by symptoms and/or to clarify abnormal outcomes of the obligatory diagnostic procedures.

IV.3 Standardisation of the diagnostic evaluation of the breast

IV.3.1 Imaging procedures

a. Mammography

Mammography is the most important imaging method in the diagnosis of breast disease. There are two types of mammographical imaging of the breast: screening mammography and diagnostic mammography.

Screening mammography is defined as the use of two-view mammography in asymptomatic women for the detection of unsuspected breast cancer [2]. In screening mammography the oblique en craniocaudal view are the standard images. Screening mammography is recommended in women over the age of 50 years.

Diagnostic mammography is a comprehensive radiological examination and consultation. In addition to the standard craniocaudal and mediolateral oblique views, the examination may include multiple specialized views, which may be indicated as part of the examination. It is performed under the direct, on-site supervision of a physician qualified in mammography. Mammography should be available for all women over the age of 35 years. The use of mammography prior to the age of 35 years is of limited diagnostic use and carries a higher risk from ionising radiation. The technical requirements of the mammography equipment are described in the European Guidelines for Quality Assurance in Mammography Screening (EUREF) [3].

All mammograms require a permanent identification label containing the name (and address) of the institution, the patient's name, a unique patient identification number and the date of the examination. Each film should be labelled left or right and the view should be specified.

The standard oblique view and the craniocaudal view must meet the criteria for good positioning described in the European Guidelines for Screening Mammography.

Definition

Oblique view

- The pectoralis muscle should be visible in the image at least to the level of the nipple
- The pectoralis muscle must angle about 20
- The glandular tissue should appear evenly spread
- The inframammary fold should be included inferiorly
- Symmetrical positioning of the images

Craniocaudal view

- Alignment of the nipple at centre or slightly medial
- Evenly spread of the glandular tissue
- Pectoralis muscle should be visible in at least 25% of the images.

In diagnostic imaging of the breast, other views can be used. Additional views are necessary in the assessment of abnormalities reported on the screening mammography examination.

The most important additional views include:

- Mediolateral or lateromedial view
- Spot compression and magnification view
- Exaggerated lateral craniocaudal view or Cleopatra view
- Rolled views

Rare applications include:

- The axillary view
- Cleavage view, for the evaluation of lesions in the internal quadrant
- Eklund view, for the evaluation of breast implants

Assessment of microcalcifications requires orthogonal projections, i.e. true lateral and cranio caudal view, and magnification views.

In order to limit unnecessary exposure to ionising radiation and discomfort of the patient because of repeated compression, the technical retake level of mammograms must preferably be below 1% and certainly not more than 3% [4].

The **mammography report** must contain the following items:

- Level of reliability based on parenchymal density
- Segmental involvement
- Description of the lesion(s): size, morphology, localisation
- Secondary malignant signs
- Conclusion of the mammographical image (BI-RADS classification [5])
- Advise and complementary examinations

If a women complaints of, or is found to have a palpable lesion or other clinical sign, she must be referred for an additional ultrasound examination, as part of the triple assessment procedure.

b. Ultrasound

After mammography, ultrasound is the most important breast imaging modality.

Because the inability to image all microcalcifications and because its very high false positive rate, ultrasound cannot be used for breast cancer screening. The examination is also very operator dependent and time consuming. Quality assurance of the technique is not established. Therefore, only members of medical staff specially trained and experienced with this procedure should carry out ultrasound.

In the assessment of abnormal clinical findings in young women (<30 years) and during pregnancy, ultrasound is usually the first imaging study in the diagnostic workup.

Until now, IBUS (International Breast Ultrasound School) proposes guidelines for the ultrasonic examination of the breast [6]. The most important indications are:

- Characterizing masses that are incompletely or not assessed by mammography
- Characterizing palpable masses
- Diagnosis of cysts
- Imaging guidance for percutaneous biopsy and localization

In the radiological protocol a BI-RADS classification or other classification can be used to summarize the results of the ultrasonic report.

Since the ultrasonography is frequently done immediately after the mammographical examination, a conclusion of both imaging techniques is necessary.

This conclusion must contain the BI-RADS (or other) classification of the lesion(s), the correct position of the lesion(s) and advises about other investigation techniques or follow up schema.

The indeterminate and suspicious lesions must undergo the process of triple assessment, i.e. besides of a clinical, and radiological examination, a cytological/histological investigation is necessary.

c. Magnetic resonance imaging

Contrast-enhanced MRI is the most sensitive additional imaging modality for evaluation of breast lesions. Due to the moderate to low specificity, MRI of the breast should be restricted to selected indications. Until now there are no guidelines for the technical requirements of MRI of the breast.

The information, coming from a MRI of the breast is based on the presence of enhancement, morphology and dynamics of enhancement. Varying interpretation rules have been suggested. These rules have an impact on the sensitivity and specificity of the examination.

To obtain the highest accuracy, it is recommended

- To consider all available MRI information
- To make the final diagnosis based on MRI **and** conventional images
- For lesions, only seen on MRI, rules which give a higher specificity are necessary, in order to avoid too many false positives.
- Technique: a dedicated breast coil should be used

The indications for an MRI investigation (in order of specificity)

- Staging of tumour extent within the breast and exclusion of multicentricity in the same or contra lateral breast
- Assessment of scarring after breast-conserving therapy (preferentially 18 months after radiation therapy)
- Evaluation after silicon implant
- Problem solving early after surgery
- Monitoring of neoadjuvant chemotherapy
- Search for primary tumour when the primary tumour is unknown and breast cancer is suspected

IV.3.2 Biopsy techniques

Via vacuum aspiration **fine needle aspiration cytology (FNAC)** sample cells, which are then cytologically analysed. A thin needle (21 gauge) is used. Samples are preferentially investigated with the thin-layer technique (Autocyte – Prep).

With **core biopsy** small tissue samples are taken out of the lesion. The thickness of the needle can be 18 G, 16 G or 14 G. Smaller needles result in less diagnostic specimen. A 14 G needle is preferred. Most systems are available in "long throw (20 mm)" and "short throw (15 mm)". Because of better tissue sampling, a long throw is preferred.

In experienced centers, both FNAC and core needle biopsy have nearly the same sensitivity (80–97%) and specificity (97–99%). The most important problem for FNAC, and less for core needle biopsy is insufficient material. The percentage of insufficient biopsies or cytology's must be lower than 10%. When FNAC is very cellular and of good technical quality, a frequent problem is the differential diagnosis between a benign proliferate lesion and a well-differentiated carcinoma.

Another problem is that some lesions frequently give a low cellular specimen (lobular carcinoma) and invasiveness is less reliable. FNAC is still very useful in the evaluation of cystic lesions and lymph nodes. Core needle biopsy is the standard method for masses, probably benign lesions and for proving malignancy in suspicious lesion. The sensitivity is much higher for masses than for microcalcifications. The value of core biopsy for the workup of architectural distortions is limited since only the positive diagnosis of malignancy is reliable.

Vacuum assisted core biopsy aspirates tissue in the needle aperture, then cuts off this aspirated tissue and moves it back in the needle where it can be collected. When the lesion is totally removed a clip must be placed and if necessary a control mammogram after the procedure must be taken. Vacuum assisted biopsy has the highest accuracy. Core biopsy underestimates more frequently ADH-DCIS and DCIS – IDA comparing with vacuum assisted core biopsy.

Vacuum assisted core biopsy is best suited for the work-up of microcalcifications, frequently done under stereotactic guidance, but ultrasonograpic guidance is also possible. When microcalcifications are biopsied (core or vacuum assisted core biopsy) a RX of the specimen is necessary in order to evaluate the biopsied calcifications and the histological results.

The radiological report of the invasive procedure must contain a description of the procedure, the amount of (core) biopsy specimen and if necessary, a description of the complications.

IV.3.3   Preoperative localization

Preoperative localization marks a non-palpable lesion, detected in a diagnostic imaging study, for subsequent excision. Non-palpable lesions must be localized with the modality that best shows the lesion (ultrasound or mammography guidance and, much less frequently, under CT or MRI guidance).

Before the procedure starts, the radiologist should review all the imaging studies. The availability of the radiological report and a true lateral and craniocaudal view is necessary. A close and clear communication with the surgeon, about the lesions that need localization, is necessary. The selection of the localization materials depends on the interval between localization and the surgery. Today, localization wires are mostly used. The distance of the tumour and the localization wire may never exceed 10 mm. If necessary, multiple needles must be placed.

All methods require documentation of the final position of the localization wire (or other material) together with a true lateral and craniocaudal view at the end of the procedure. The radiological protocol must contain a description of the procedure and of the localization of the needle related to the lesion. Correct excision of the non-palpable lesion should always be documented by specimen radiography or sometimes specimen sonography where necessary. If possible the specimen must be X-rayed in two positions in order to better evaluate the margins.

IV.4 Prognostic and predictive factors

Introduction

Besides classical markers such as TNM and markers for proliferation, a large number of tumour-associated biomarkers have been tested to better predict outcome and result of therapy in breast cancer. Only a few markers yield sufficiently validated, statistically independent prognostic and/or predictive value and can be measured in clinical routine with quality control. At this time, only steroid hormone receptor status, Her-2 status and certain components (uPA, PAI-1) of the plasminogen activator system are considered for routine use.

IV.4.1 ER and PgR: methods and definitions

The level of receptors for the steroid hormones estradiol (ER) and/or progesterone (PgR) in tumour tissue is a strong indicator of the extent of hormone dependency of breast cancer. Both markers, ER and PgR, are largely used in clinical practice to select, for each patient individually, the most appropriate form of systemic adjuvant or palliative endocrine therapy.

Within the context of clinical trials, ER and PgR are widely used either as stratification criteria before randomisation, or to select patient populations likely to benefit from hormonal manipulations. In advanced disease the presence ER and PgR is correlated with a better clinical outcome. Receptor-positive tumours are frequently better differentiated, and have lower proliferation rates than receptor-negative lesions.

Assays

(a) The classical biochemical assay (Ligand Binding Assay, LBA)

ER and PgR are proteins, which bind with high affinity and great specificity estradiol–17β (E2) and progesterone (Pg), respectively. Measuring the binding capacity of ER and PgR for tritiated steroids in tumour tissue homogenates can identify them. After ultra-centrifugation, ER and PgR are generally present in the cytosol (supernatant) and in the nuclear fraction (pellet), but for practical reasons, most laboratories run their assays on the cytosol only. This cytosol fraction is subsequently incubated with different concentrations of tritiated estradiol or with a tritiated progesterone derivate. Unbound steroids are subsequently removed by the addition of a Dextran-Coated Charcoal suspension, followed by centrifugation (DCC method). Binding capacity of the receptors for the steroids is calculated using Scatchard analysis. The receptor concentration is expressed as fmol/mg tissue extract protein. This assay has been standardised by the EORTC Receptor and Biomarker Group. An external trans-European quality assessment scheme, already running for more than 20 years, still monitors the performance of participating laboratories.

(b) The enzyme Immuno Assay (EIA)

Monoclonal antibodies to ER and PgR, respectively, have been produced, which allow specific recognition of the ER and PgR antigen. These monoclonal antibodies allow recognition of the receptors even when their ligand binding sites are occupied by steroid hormones or synthetic analogues. As in the cytosol fraction, ER is predominantly present in the unoccupied form, the quantitative results obtained with the EIA are almost identical to those given by the LBA method. While the LBA method in general requires at least 100 mg tissue to yield valid results, the EIA can be reliably performed on tissue samples weighing 50 mg or less.

(c) Immuno Histo-/-Cytochemical Assay (IHA-/-ICA)

Monoclonal antibodies, including those used for the EIA, have been developed for immuno-staining of histologically and (-cytologically-) identifiable tumour cells. The semi-quantitative results of the IHA/ICA are in acceptable concordance with those of the LBA and EIA techniques.

The major drawback of this technique is related to the lack of standardization regarding fixation and staining, and of the different ways of scoring of the results, which have to take into account the intensity of staining of individual cells and the number of cells stained. Still, the method is simple and widely accessible. Moreover, ER and PgR determinations can be done in fresh and paraffin embedded tissue applying commercially available antibodies. Results of IHA/ICA's should be given a semi quantitative score according to evaluated and published scoring systems.

Phenotypes and concentration of steroid hormone receptors in tumours

The results of ER and PgR assays can be expressed either qualitatively (positive or negative status) or quantitatively (exact concentration). The EORTC Receptor and Biomarker Group (RBG) has defined that all tumours containing 10 or more fmol of ER or PgR per mg of protein should be considered as positive, although the actual content can reach values as high as 2000 fmol/mg protein. Tumours with an ER or PgR content <10 fmol/mg protein should be considered as negative. Applying these cut-off values, the distribution of ER/PgR in pre- and postmenopausal patients with newly diagnosed primary breast cancer has been assessed [Table 1]. In general, receptor positivity will decline during the course of breast cancer disease. High levels of ER and PgR are related with highest response rates to endocrine manipulations.

Table 1: ER/PgR status in breast cancer (biochemical assays).

Phenotype distribution in primary tumours	ER−/PgR−	ER−/PgR+	ER+/PgR−	ER+/PgR+
In premenopause	22%	12%	13%	52%
In postmenopause	23%	1%	35%	41%
Response rates in advanced disease	<10%	32%	40%	73%

Practical recommendations

Technique of assay
1. Because of the high thermolability of the steroid hormone receptors, the tumour tissue to be assessed should be frozen as soon as possible (preferentially within 30 minutes from excision) and without fixation after inspection by a pathologist.
2. For LBA and EIA, tumour samples should be processed according to the instructions published by the EORTC Receptor and Biomarker Group [7]. Additionally, the laboratory should be advised to participate in the quality control scheme organised by this group.
3. Both the LBA and the EIA techniques are clinically relevant for prognostic and thera-peutic purposes, and yield almost similar results. The latter (EIA) should be preferred in case of small tissue samples (<100 mg) or when receptor occupancy by an (anti) hormone is suspected. The use of the anti-estrogen tamoxifen should be withdrawn for at least 6 weeks before the tumour specimen can be excised for determination of ER and/or PgR by the LBA. Leftover, unused cytosols should be stored in a proper way ($<-70°$C freezer or in liquid nitrogen) to allow determination of other tumor-associated factors.

Interpretation of results of LBA and EIA

- The hormonal context (current or recent (anti) hormonal treatment; menopausal status) should be taken into account, since it may affect ER and PgR levels.
- Tumours containing <10 fmol ER- or PgR/mg protein should be considered as ER- or PgR negative.
- If one chooses to use the results qualitatively, the ER- or PgR-status (positive or negative) of both receptors together should be considered. The sole category of cases presumed to be almost totally hormone-independent concerns the ER-/PgR- phenotype. In this category, the chance of response to hormonal manipulations in advanced breast disease is only 10% or even lower.
- If one wants to select a highly hormone-responsive population of patients (for example with the aim of testing a new hormonal treatment, minimising the risk of beta error), one may include ER+/PgR+ cases (qualitative selection), for whom the chances of response to hormonal manipulations are close to 75%; alternatively, one may select those patients with very high ER content (>100 fmol/mg protein for postmenopausal patients; >50 fmol/mg protein for premenopausal patients), in general also displaying a positive PgR status.

Interpretation of results of IHA/ICA

- The ER and PgR status should be determined according to the scoring system which is in use at the particular hospital. There is also a need for standardisation of the assay. As long as this is not the case, values generated in one laboratory cannot be compared to those generated in another laboratory. Consequently, universal cut-off points cannot be given.
- Results of biochemical assays (LBA/EIA) and IHA/ICA's are complementary, especially when receptor negativity has to be confirmed.

In summary

- Determination of ER and PgR status is part of the routine diagnostic work-up of tumour tissue of patients operated for primary or advanced breast cancer.
- ER or PgR can be determined by LBA, EIA or IHA/ICA, as long as in a particular hospital the chosen assay is validated and quality-controlled.
- Biochemical and immunohisto-/cytochemical assays yield complementary information.
- Leftover cytosol fractions and unprocessed tumour tissues should be stored in the frozen state to allow future analysis of other tumour tissue-associated factors.

IV.4.2 Her-2

Her-2 belongs to the epidermal growth factor receptor family. Amplification of the Her-2 gene will result in overexpression of this type of receptor. In general, overexpression of Her-2 is correlated with unfavourable tumour characteristics as high mitotic index, aneuploidy and absence of steroid hormone receptor positivity, and clinically with nodal metastasis, short disease-free survival and relative resistance to therapy. Administration of a humanized, monoclonal antibody (trastuzumab; Herceptin®) against Her-2 affects Her-2 tyrosine kinase activity resulting in decreased signal transduction and cell proliferation.

Techniques of assay

A very reliable technique to detect Her-2 amplification in fixed tumour tissue sections is fluorescence in situ hybridisation (FISH). With this technique, labelled Her-2 containing DNA probes are hybridised with tumour chromosomes in a tumour section mounted on a microscope slide, allowing counting the number of Her-2 genes per involved chromosome. Other techniques include semi-quantitative immunohistochemical (IHC) detection of Her-2 expression in fixed tumour tissue specimens, for which commercially available tests are available. Results are expressed as negative, or 1+ to 3+ in which IHC 3+ is considered as Her-2 positive for clinical purposes. FISH is not routinely performed as the primary test. It usually serves as back up to select Her-2 overexpressing tumors in patients with intermediate staining at IHC (i.e. IHC 2+). It has been documented recently that results of Her-2 testing in primary tumour tissue correlates well with those determined in metastasis.

Interpretation and recommendation

In patients with advanced breast cancer, overexpression of Her-2 (IHC 3+ or FISH positive) will indicate a favourable response to treatment with trastuzumab whether or not combined with chemotherapy. Other claims, i.e. relative resistance to CMF-like (adjuvant) chemotherapy and tamoxifen treatment as well as improved outcome of adjuvant trastuzumab treatment (especially when combined with doxorubicin or taxanes) have to be confirmed.

With this in mind, routine measurement of the tumour Her-2 status as part of the clinical work-up in breast cancer is advocated, for later guiding possible palliative therapy and for estimated near future use in decision making around adjuvant treatment. Furthermore, routine determination will allow translational research about this topic in a lot of clinical studies and results may serve as an inclusion or exclusion criterion for particular clinical trials.

IV.4.3 Components of the urokinase plasminogen activator system

High tumour levels of both, urokinase-type plasminogen activator (uPA) and its inhibitor plasminogen activator inhibitor type-1 (PAI-1), correlate with increased metastasising potency and subsequent decreased disease-free and overall survival of patients with node-positive or node-negative primary breast cancer. Especially in node-negative disease, high levels of uPA and/or PAI-1 independently predict an up to 3.9 times higher relapse rate than patients with low levels of those components [8].

Assay

Commercially available ELISA assays in use are quality-controlled by the EORTC Receptor and Biomarker Group. uPA and PAI-1 are determined in extracts of frozen tumour tissue samples.

Interpretation and recommendation

Especially in node-negative breast cancer, high levels of uPA and/or PAI-1 predict for a poor outcome and should be considered as a rationale for the recommendation of adjuvant systemic therapy. The prognostic impact of these markers allows them to be ranked at the highest level of evidence, category 1. Furthermore, routine determination of uPA and PAI-1 will allow translational research to further establish their prognostic power and also their predictive (therapy response) capacities. Such results may even serve as inclusion or exclusion criteria for particular clinical trials.

Nevertheless, at presence, the scarce availability of fresh frozen tumour tissue is of disadvantage, as the ELISA cannot be done on fixed tissue. Otherwise, the uPA and PAI-1 ELISA are easy to perform, ready to be introduced into the clinic for routine determination of these promising factors in breast cancer patients.

References

1a. UICC/TNM Classification of malignant tumours. Sixth edition 2002 – Wiley-Liss.
1b. Revision of the American Joint Committee on Cancer Staging System for Breast Cancer (*J Clin Oncol*, 2002; 20:3628–36).
2. American Cancer Society ACR Bulletin 48(10):27,1992.
3. www.euref.org.
4. Perry NM; EUSOMA Working Party. Quality assurance in the diagnosis of breast disease. EUSOMA Working Party. *Eur J Cancer*. 2001 Jan;37(2):159–72.
5. Breast Imaging Reporting and Data System® Atlas BI-RADS, 4th edition (www.acr.org).
6. European Journal of Ultrasound: 9 (1999) (www.ibus.org)
7. EORTC Breast Cancer Cooperative Group. *Eur J Cancer* 1980;16:1513–15.
8. Look MP, van Putten WL, Duffy MJ, Harbeck N et al. Pooled analysis of prognostic impact of urokinase-type plasminogen activator and its inhibitor PAI-1 in 8377 breast cancer patients. *J Natl Cancer Inst.* 2002 Jan 16;94(2):116–28.

V. Pathology

V.1 Introduction

The next paragraphs provide the preferred methods for pathologists for the handling and reporting of breast surgery specimens.

Molecular biologic techniques, requiring fresh-frozen tumor tissue, will be increasingly used to provide prognostic and predictive information. It is therefore necessary that all specimens are delivered immediately, unfixed and intact to the laboratory.

V.2 Handling open diagnostic biopsy specimen

An open diagnostic biopsy is performed when a diagnosis was not obtained by non-operative procedures (fine needle biopsy and/or core biopsy). Most cases concern mammographically detected non-palpable lesions. Work-up of these lesions requires radiology guided evaluation with a specimen X-ray in toto to assess the representativity of the surgical biopsy, and a X-ray of the lamellated specimen to facilitate selection of tissue for histologic studies.

Histologic evaluation requires optimal slides, and often extensive sampling and use of immuno-histochemical stainings. Frozen section for the diagnosis of these lesions is inappropriate. All diagnostic biopsy specimens should be handled as if the procedure was part of breast conserving surgery (see V.3).

V.3 Handling of therapeutic wide local excision (breast conserving surgery)

It is not possible to orientate the specimen without surgical guidance; request surgeons for necessary information, especially

– side
– quadrant location
– orientation of nipple and deep surface with long and short sutures.

* *Record* specimen size in 3 dimensions in cm, and weight.

* *Mark* margins with Indian ink using a protocol with different colours to enable recognition of different surfaces in slides. Ink will adhere well when fresh specimen are blotted free of blood and moisture, or when specimen are dipped in methanol or 10% acetic acid for a few seconds.

* Make *serial sections* at 0.3–0.5 cm intervals perpendicular to the nipple-periphery axis.

* *Cooling* the specimen wrapped in aluminium-foil for 20' at −20°C facilitates sectioning.

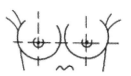 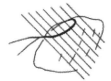

* *Record*
– largest diameter grossly identifiable tumor
– aspect of tumor features (round, stellate, irregular etc.)
– minimal distances from surgical edges. Frozen section studies of margins is discouraged unless the tumor seems to be close to a margin and preoperative conformation of this will have immediate impact on treatment.

* Select tumor tissue for fresh-frozen tumor banking.

* Fixate the slices flat between gauzes for 24 hours in 6% neutral buffered formalin.

(Optional: make X-ray of serial sections; a specimen X-ray is helpful to assess tumor distribution and relation with margins, and when preoperative mammography reports the presence of microcalcifications. Good quality X-rays can be made when the slices are blotted free of moisture).

* *Sample* for microscopy.
– complete cross-section of tumor at the level of the largest diameter including periphery and surrounding tissue
– macroscopic nearest surgical edges
– all grossly or radiological abnormal tissue from remaining specimen

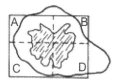 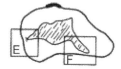

V.4 Handling excision biopsy specimen; DCIS and M. Paget

DCIS

Surgical tretment of DCIS requires a complete excision with free margins. Assessment of margins of excision requires careful pathologic study.

Generally, the *first biopsy* is a *diagnostic procedure*. The pathologic examination should be focussed on the diagnosis of DCIS, and exclusion of invasive growth. As rule of thumb, all tissue should be embedded or, in larger specimen, at least 8 blocks containing DCIS, to exclude invasive growth.

A *second wide re-excision* is often necessary to achieve a complete excision. Pathologic work-up should follow the manual for excision biopsy specimen (V.3). Whenever possible, a radiography of the lamellated specimen in sequential ordered slices should be obtained to pinpoint areas with microcalcifications. All grossly and/or radiologically abnormal areas should be sampled. Breast tissue surrounding the biopsy site, tissue nearest to the nipple and the periphery should be extensively sampled. The specimen X-ray is extremely useful to mark the sites from which the blocks are taken.

M. Paget

The specimen consists of a central cone biopsy with skin and (part of) the nipple areola. The surgeon should mark the 12-o'clock site on the skin. The nipple areola should be totally sampled in sequential transverse sections. The 12-o'clock site can be marked in the sections with a small skin incision.

For the breast cone the manual for excision biopsy specimen should be followed (V.3). The specimen should be preferably sectioned in slices giving transverse sections, perpendicular to the main ducts. Whenever possible, X-rays of the section in sequential order should be obtained to pinpoint microcalcifications and select areas for microscopic study.

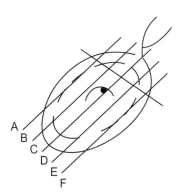

V.5   Handling of mastectomy specimen

* Ask the surgeon to indicate the 12-o'clock point on the skin, for instance with a suture, and to give necessary information about side, and quadrant location of the tumor.

* Record the size of the specimen, dimensions and appearance of the skin, appearance and location of the nipple, site of previous biopsy if present. Record whether the pectoral fascia is intact and the presence of pectoral muscle.

* Section the specimen at 0.5–1 cm intervals, preferably through the posterior surface up to the skin, perpendicular to the 12- and 6-o'clock axis. Place the macrosegments in sequential order.

* Describe tumor, if present, in the same way as in the excisional biopsy specimen (V.3). The size and relation to the surgical margins of a biopsy site should be recorded, and the presence, location and size of residual tumor. The minimum distances from the skin, surgical edges and deep tissues should be noted.

* Sample tumor tissue for fresh-frozen tissue banking

* Fixate the slices flat between gauzes for 24 hours in 6% neutral buffered formalin.

* Sample for microscopy:

- a full cross-section from the grossly identifiable tumor including its periphery and surrounding tissue, if necessary in more than one block.
- blocks from skin, fascia and pectoral muscle if the tumor is close to these.
- all grossly suspicious lesions, and at least one tissue block from each quadrant.
- a section of the subareolar region perpendicular to the main ducts.

V.6 Handling of axillary lymph nodes and sentinel nodes

Axillary lymph node specimen

The axillary lymph nodes are received "en bloc" with the breast or as a separate specimen in case of breast conserving treatment.

The three axillary lymph node levels can only be distinguished in radical mastectomy specimens. In the other specimens only inner and outer axillary tail nodes can be distinguished from basal nodes. Therefore, the surgeon should mark the inner and outer axillary tail in the mastectomy specimen, and both axillary tail and breast side (for instance with long, short and double sutures) in separate axillary specimens.

All nodes from inner, outer and lowest part of the specimen should be sampled in 3 portions. The nodes should be totally embedded. Nodes up to 0.5 cm can be completely embedded, several per block; nodes from 0.5 to 1 cm should be bisected and embedded separately, one node per block. Nodes larger than 1 cm should be embedded in serial sections of 2–3 mm, if necessary in multiple blocks.

At least 10 lymph nodes should be obtained. Lymph node dissection done in fresh specimen by palpation may yield the highest number of nodes.

The number of nodes should be recorded. Lymph node aggregates fixed to one another should be noted. Gross involvement with metastases should be recorded.

Routine work-up of axillary nodes includes one level sections and HE staining. Step sections and immunostaining with keratin antibodies has been shown to result in the detection of mainly micro-metastases with a questionable prognostic significance; use of these methods is therefore not mandated in routine clinical practice.

Sentinel node (SN) procedure

Axillary lymph node staging by the SN procedure is increasingly performed. There is no consensus what the best method is to assess the SN node status. The chance to detect metastases correlates with to what proportion the node is studied. The chance on metastases in the remaining axillary nodes increases with the amount of tumor deposits in the SN. In accordance with the TNM classification these are classified as macrometastases (>2 mm), micrometastases (0.2–2 mm), and submicrometastases (<0.2 mm), or isolated tumor cells (ITC). In the TNM classification micrometastases are considered metastases, and deposits <0.2 mm are not. The aim of SN evaluation should therefore be directed on the detection of deposits ≥0.2 mm. This can be achieved by step sectioning SN's with 200 micron distance. It is practical to use 3 to 5 levels per paraffin block (meaning 6–10 levels of a bisected node). Adding more levels, and use of immunohistochemistry will increase the detection rate of submicrometastases, and therefore reduces practicality of SN assessment; these methods may be used in research and trial settings.

Routine handling of SN's: Lymph nodes larger than 4 mm should be bisected; larger than 10 mm completely embedded in 2–3 mm thick sections.

Preoperative frozen section study may be requested; only one level of the sections should then be used for the frozen section procedure; all the residual material should be examined by paraffin sections.

Definite histopathologic examination of the SN should be based on at least 3 step sections of the paraffin blocks, with at least 150 and maximally 250 microns intervals; sections should be stained by HE (optional: cytokeratins (8 and 18, CAM 5.2)).

V.7 Reporting of breast specimens

The complete pathologic report on a breast specimen should provide the clinicians all data for optimal adjuvant treatment planning and treatment evaluation in future.

The full pathology report includes:

a. Clinical information

- side, quadrant location, appropriate details from preoperative studies (physical examination, mammography, aspiration cytology or gross needle biopsy)
- type of specimen.

b. Macroscopic findings

- size of specimen in 3 dimensions, largest diameter grossly identifiable tumor (pT), and relations to nearest surgical edges, skin or deep tissues.
- number of lymph nodes separately in inner and outer top levels and basal portions. Presence of lymph nodes fixed to one another.

c. Microscopic findings

(1) Tumor type
(2) Microscopic distribution of both invasive and non-invasive parts of the tumor
(3) Tumor grade
(4) Microscopic relation to surgical edges
(5) Vascular invasion
(6) SN status/lymph node status (pN)
(7) Immunohistochemical steroid receptor status (optional Her-2 status)
(8) Additional

ad. 1. *Tumor type*. Tumors should be classified according the WHO criteria (Tumors of the Breast, Lyon 2003, IARC press). Mixtures of different types in the same tumor mass should be recorded separately. "Uncertain" or "unclassifiable" tumors should be recorded as such.

For *in situ* lesions the histologic classification designed by the EORTC pathology working party of the breast group should be used, as described in Seminars in Diagnostic Pathology 1994, Vol 11, No 3, pages 167–180.

ad. 2. Growth pattern (expansive vs. invasive; unifocal vs. multinodular or diffuse) should be recorded. The pT should be adjusted when the microscopic tumor size exceeds gross measurement. Satellite lesions should not be included in pT measurement, diffuse growth around a dominant lesion (as in ILC may be found) should.

When present, the DCIS component surrounding an invasive tumor should be recorded; its amount and extent and relation to margins should be evaluated and (semi)quantitated. As a rule of thumb, an extensive DCIS component requires involvement of 10 ductulo-lobular units.

In case of pure DCIS the extent should be measured by radiology–histology correlation. Usually the microscopic extent exceeds the radiologic area of microcalcifications.

ad. 3. The Bloom and Richardson grading system as adapted by Elston and Ellis should be used (Histopatholoy 1991; 19: 403–410).

ad. 4. *Assessment of margins.* Tumor transsected at an inked surface represents clearly involved margins. Margin involvement should be specified (invasive and/or *in situ* carcinoma), (semi)quantified (focal = area of less than 3 mm, or extensive), and located (nipple side/ basal side, etc.).

For DCIS treated with excision biopsy the best guarantee of completeness appears to be when unifocal DCIS is surrounded by normal glandular breast tissue or a margin of at least 1 cm uninvolved tissue, or when a re-excision specimen contains no tumor.

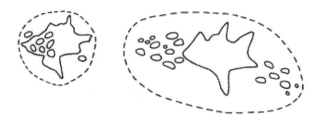

ad. 5. *Vascular invasion.* Tumor emboli should be found in at least 3 endothelium-lined vessels in tissue surrounding the tumor.

ad. 6. pN. UICC guidelines for classification of SN and axillary nodes should be followed (TNM Supplement, UICC, Third Edition, Wiley–Liss, 2003).

ad. 7. Immunohistochemical steroid receptor (and Her-2) status assessment. Laboratories assessing these receptors should prove the sensitivity and specificity of their methods by internal and external quality assurance. Analyses should preferably on slides containing normal glandular breast tissue as internal control. In-house controls should come from composite blocks containing receptor rich, receptor poor, an receptor negative tumors. Laboratories must take part in a regular external quality assurance scheme.

Reporting the results of steroid receptor immunohistochemistry can best be done by giving the percentage of staining nuclei. DAKO criteria should be used for Her-2 evaluation.

ad. 8. Additional features may be added individually at different laboratories. For evaluation of some of the EORTC Breast Cancer Group trials, slides are reviewed by the EORTC breast pathology panel.

d. Conclusion

Type of specimen (side), tumor type, grade, size (maximum diameter, pT), margin status. SN/axillary node status; total number, number and location of involved nodes (pN).

VI.   The sentinel node biopsy

VI.1 Definition

The sentinel node (SN) is the first lymph node on a direct drainage pathway from the primary tumour site; the tumour site may drain to more than one sentinel lymph node.

VI.2   Techniques of identification

Three techniques are studied to identify the SN:

1. Lymphoscintigraphy after injection of a radioactive tracer
2. The intraoperative use of a gamma probe after injection of a radioactive tracer.
3. Injection of patent blue dye with intraoperative mapping by following blue lymphatics into blue sentinel lymph nodes.

The optimal technique as to where to inject the tracer has not yet been established. Relative controversies exists about:

− volume of colloid (varying between 0.2 and 6 ml)
− type of colloid (Nanocoll, Albures, Sulphur Colloid)
− volume of Patent Blue dye
− type of blue dye (Patent Blue dye, Lymphazurin)
− location of injection: into the tumour, peritumorally, subcutaneously, intracutaneously over the tumour site, or intracutaneously peri-areolar.

A number of directions are becoming clear:

− Patent Blue dye works good, is cheap and widely available in Europe.
− Intra- or peritumoral injection of a radioactive tracer followed by lymfoscintigraphy leads frequently (up to 20%) to sentinel nodes apart from the axilla (internal mammary chain, intramammary, intrapectoral, infraclavicular).
− Sub- or ultracutaneous injection results in a swift flow to the axilla and therefore higher identification rates (by higher uptake) in the axilla, however only rarely to other sites.
− After injection of Patent Blue dye, massage of the breast improves flow, facilitating the identification of blue lymphatics and nodes more easily.
− Lymphoscintigraphy with dynamic (first thirty minutes after the injection) and static (after 2 and 4 hours) facilitates the differentiation between sentinel nodes and non-sentinel nodes, and the identification of the sentinel node in- and outside the axilla. If lymphoscintigraphy shows sentinel nodes, identification is in almost 100% of the patients possible.
− The use of a sensitive probe during surgery facilitates identification of sentinel node (particularly in obese patients and when Patent Blue dye fails).
− Patent Blue dye improves the identification rate. It can be used when lymphoscintigraphy does not show drainage (in about 10–15%), and during surgery. Sometimes blue nodes are identified which are not radioactive.
− The combined technique is very helpful in the learning phase and has been shown to result in the highest identification rates (>95% after 50 cases).
− In general the combined technique including lymphoscintigraphy, intraoperative use of the gamma probe and lymphatic mapping by Patent Blue dye is recommended (when available).
− Technetium colloid is easily retained in the SN, does not migrate and gamma ray activity remains sufficient till 36 hours post injection. This enables to perform lymphoscintigraphy the day before surgery.
− Surgery is performed between 2 to 36 hours after injection of radioactive tracer.

VI.3 Surgery

Just before sterile draping the blue dye is injected (1–4 cc; in or around the tumour, intracutaneously). The location of the SN is identified by scanning with the probe over the site where the SN's are suspected (and preferably indicated by the nuclear physician according to the lymphoscintigraphy). After massaging the breast (for a few minutes), the incision is placed over the location were the sentinel node is suspected.

If the sentinel node is in the axilla, the incision is usually placed behind the free edge of the major pectoral muscle at the lower border of the hair implant. The blue lymphatics can usually be identified behind Scarpas fascia. The dissection should be meticulous, not to sever the lymphatics. If no blue lymphatics are identifed, the probe can be used to identify the radioactive nodes. Radioactive and/or blue nodes are removed and afferent or efferent lymphatics secured.

Internal mammary chain nodes can be approached either by a separate incision or through the same incision for mastectomy or wide local excision. The identification and removal of the SN is at the medial site of the intercostal space along the internal mammary artery. It requires careful dissection, but it is not a difficult technique. All nodes that are possibly SN are removed (if lymphoscintigraphy shows unequivocally non SN or second echelon SN, these hot nodes are not to be removed).

VI.4 Learning phase

- The sentinel node technique requires careful logistic and technical processing with a close co-operation between surgeon, nuclear physician and pathologist.
- It is mandatory to attend a training course by all members of the team (particularly surgeon and nuclear physician).
- In general after 25 to 35 procedures under guidance or with confirmational lymph node dissection (ALND) the identification rate remains over 90%. After 50 cases, the identification rate is usually over 95%.

VI.5   Current status

-   The SN-concept in breast cancer has proven to be valid.
-   With experience the identification rate of SN is over 95%.
-   The false negative rate (missing a tumour positive axilla by a tumour negative sentinel node) is reported to be 3 to 5% in experienced hands after confirmational axillary lymph node dissection.
-   Clinical false negative rate after omitting full ALND in case of a tumour negative SN is reported to be less than 2% after follow-up of 3–4 years.
-   The sentinel node procedure will lead to upstaging as a result of the more careful histologic work up of the sentinel nodes (those nodes which are most likely to harbour metastasis) and examination of nodes which would otherwise not be found or removed.
-   In experienced hands, the sentinel node procedure in invasive breast cancer can be considered as an equal staging procedure as ALND.
-   The clinical relevance of micrometastasis found by immunohistochemistry (single cells), or tumour tracers by RT-PCR technique is unknown.
-   The chance of finding more tumour positive nodes if the sentinel node is tumour positive, varies between 10 to 50% (from a number of published series). If the sentinel node contains micrometastasis (smaller than 2 mm), the chance for more positive nodes is published to be between 10 and 30%.
-   Treatment of the axilla is advised if the sentinel node is tumour positive.

VI.6   Indications

The highest identification rates are maintained when:

- lymphoscintigraphy is positive
- when both lymphoscintigraphy, probe and Patent Blue dye is applied
- the personal experience is over 50 procedures
- after intradermal injection, the identification rate of the axilla is the best
- if no upfront chemotherapy or radiotherapy is applied
- if no wide excision has been performed.

The lowest false negative rate is expected when:

- the lymphoscintigraphy is positive
- the sentinel nodes are definitively identified (radioactive, blue. combined, blue lymphatics into a blue lymph node)
- the invasive part of the tumour is less than 3 to 4 cm without a previous wide local excision.

A diagnostic excision of the invasive tumour appears not to result in lower identification rates.

VII. Primary treatment: surgery

VII.1   Definitions

VII.2   Minimal requirements for documentation in the operation report by the surgeon

VII.3   Minimal requirements for information from surgeon to pathologist

VII.1 Definitions

The descriptions are based on clinical and/or preoperative judgement and are irrespective of pathology findings.

In all operative specimens marker signs should be applied to facilitate an exact pathological assessment of the extent of the disease.

This should be discussed in detail with the pathologists (see VII.3).

Localization titanium clips should be left in the excision cavity to aid in placement of irradiation boost volume.

It is strongly recommended to perform a control mammography to confirm that no micro-calcifications remain in patients in whom microcalcification-containing breast tissue is removed for diagnosis or therapeutic reasons in case of malignancy.

a. Incisional biopsy

Only part of the tumor is excised; a macroscopic residue is left in the patient.

b. Excisional biopsy (tumorectomy)

Excision without margins but with the intention of removing all clinically suspicious tissue with a surrounding cuff of normal tissue. Palpation of the operation cavity should not disclose abnormalities.

c. Lumpectomy (wide local excision)

Excision of tumor with an estimated 1 cm margin of (macroscopically) normal breast tissue around the lesion.

Palpation of the operation cavity should not disclose any abnormality. Overlying skin can be removed for cosmetic or oncological reasons. The margins may be smaller in the direction of the muscles; in case of this margin being less than 1 cm, the muscle fascia should be carefully included in the operation. The deepest point might be marked with a clip; the type of clip should be discussed with the radiology department.

d. Partial or segmental mastectomy

The tumor is removed at least with 2 cm margin of apparently normal tissue. This procedure usually involves removing less tissue than a quadrantectomy but more than a lumpectomy. The skin can be removed for cosmetic or oncological reasons. The margins may be smaller in the direction of the muscles; in case of this margin being less than 1 cm, the muscle fascia should be carefully included in the operation. The deepest point might be marked with a clip; the type of clip should be discussed with the radiology department.

e. Quadrantectomy

Removal of about 2 cm portion of normal mammary tissue around the tumor, together with portions of overlying skin and underlying pectoral fascia by means of a radial incision defining a cone-shaped excision piece.

f.   Skin-sparing mastectomy

Removal of the entire breast with preservation of its skin, except the nipple and the areola to facilitate immediate reconstruction. Skin sparing mastectomy should only be performed in the contest of immediate reconstruction.

g.   Total (simple) mastectomy

Removal of the entire breast with its skin and the nipple-areola complex, with the pectoralis major muscle fascia, but without axillary node dissection.

h.   Modified radical mastectomy

1.   type Madden:
   –   en bloc removal of the complete breast and the axilla; for the extent of axillary clearance (see VII.1.l).
2.   type Patey:
   –   as h.1. but including resection of m. pectoralis minor.

i.   Radical mastectomy (type "Halsted")

As h.2. but including resection of (part of) sternal part of the m. pectoralis major.

j.   Image directed surgery

Nonpalpable carcinoma could be diagnosed by image-directed microbiopsy or localization biopsy procedure. Before definitive surgery localization procedures are mandatory. The target is full excision of the tumor with uniform margin. Hook wire, blue dye injection, or radioguided occult lesion localization (ROLL) are the standard approaches. The latter method is useful also for sentinel lymph node biopsy. The localization will be facilitated by the placement of a marker clip when image guided biopsy is done for small lesions, which are likely to be completely removed by the procedure. After excision a specimen radiography, preferably in two projections, is performed to verify the excision of the lesion.

k.   Microdochectomy, cone biopsy

The removal through a curved perimamillary or small radial incision of a single, or all (cone biopsy) of the milk ducts from beneath the nipple which may be associated with nipple discharge. Patent blue staining is the method of choice to facilitate accurate minimal volume of resection. The excision specimen is marked near the nipple (e.g. by sutures).

l.   Axillary clearance (axillary dissection)

–   All incisions are acceptable, providing there has been sufficient exposure of the entire axillary content;
–   In breast conservation cases the clearance should preferably be performed discontinuously from the breast excision using transverse incisions;
–   All axillary fat from at least levels I and II should be excised in one specimen;
–   The medial border is formed by a curved plane ranging from the muscles to the vessels and nerves going to the pectoral muscles (in the interpectoral area, the interpectoral fat, which might contain nodes, should be dissected carefully from this neurovascular bundles). The medial line is further indicated by a sagittal plane through the medial border of the m. pectoralis minor (patient in supine position).

- The cranial border is formed by plexus and axillary vein;
- The lateral border is from the white tendon downward to the m. latissimus dorsi;
- The dorsal border is the fascia of subscapular muscles; the n. thoracodorsalis and vessels may be spared, but should be resected in cases with suspicious nodes fixed to these structures;
- Caudally the upper-outer quadrant of the breast; care is given to resect the fat between thoracic wall and upper-outer quadrant of the breast; resection of parts of breast tissue might therefore be necessary;
- The m. pectoralis minor may be resected;
- Level III axillary fat (apical, subclavicular) may be resected, en bloc with the specimen or separately for staging procedures.

m. Node sampling

Picking out at least four individual (suspected) axillary lymph nodes usually located in the lower part of the axilla. This procedure is not recommended because of the possibility of sampling error (inadequate diagnosis) and irradicality (inadequate therapy).

n. Infraclavicular (apical) biopsy (Haagensen)

This is an optional staging procedure. Some institutes perform an apical biopsy in all operable breast cancer cases, others only in higher stage breast cancer. The space limited by the subclavian vein cranially, the medial border of the minor pectoral muscle laterally, the thoracic wall dorsally and medially, and the inferior pectoral fascia ventrally is considered to contain level III lymph nodes. Clearance of this space is called apical biopsy or level III clearance.

o. Sentinel node (SN) biopsy

This procedure is being used to select clinically node-negative patients for treatment of the axilla. Both dye injected at the tumor site, transported to the first (sentinel) node and radioactive tracers have to be used to optimally locate the sentinel node (see chapter VI).

The operative field of the SN biopsy should be as small as possible, creating the maximal possibility to remove the SN as the only target, minimizing implantation risk. The SN is incidentally not localized in the base of the axilla (but in IM node or in the infraclavicular or Rotter area); tumor positive findings in these locations have specific therapeutic implications.

p. Level I dissection of the axilla

This staging procedure is performed by some institutes in T1N0 lesions to assess axillary involvement. The axillary content lateral from the minor pectoral muscle is removed.

q. Internal mammary node biopsy

This staging procedure is performed by some institutes to investigate internal mammary node involvement. The intercostal muscles in the medial parts of the second (and third) intercostal space(s) are divided. Fatty tissue around the internal mammary vessels is removed. The parietal pleura is preserved.

VII.2   Minimal requirements for documentation in the operation report by the surgeon

To be able to compare operation techniques and results, the surgeon is advised to report the following aspects of breast surgery.

a.   In local breast excision

- Whether the removal of the tumor is considered to be excisional (with no or very small margins), a lumpectomy (margin about 1 cm), or segment-/quadrantectomy (margin 2 cm or more).
- Whether the basal fascia has been reached, incised or excised
- Whether the breast tissue and/or subcutis has been closed by sutures (type, degradable material).
- Whether a drain has been placed
- Used localization technique
- Whether an x-ray (one or two projections) of the specimen has been done and the result
- If and how a so called oncoplastic procedure has been performed
- Whether localization clips have been left in the tumor bed

b.   In node biopsies

- Exact location
- Used localization technique (in sentinel node biopsy)

c.   In axillary dissection

- Level I, II or III dissection, especially whether the top of the specimen is level II (nodes dorsal from the minor pectoral muscle) or level III (nodes medial from pectoral minor muscle)
- Whether the thoraco-dorsal neuro-vascular bundle has been spared or sacrificed
- Whether the larger thoracic nerve has been spared
- Whether the intercostobrachial nerves have been spared
- Whether the minor pectoral muscle has been spared
- Clinical aspects of lymph nodes (e.g. whether suspected of containing metastasis or whether the excision was macroscopically radical)

d.   In ablative surgery

- Type of incision (periareolar, horizontal, oblique, vertical)
- Type of mastectomy:
  "Skin sparing mastectomy" (VII.1.f)
  "Madden" (VII.1.h1)
  "Patey" (VII.1.h2)
  "Halsted" (VII.1.i)
  Type of axillary clearance
  Levels I + II
  Levels I + II + III
- Whether the longer thoracic and dorsal thoracic nerves have been spared
- The use and number of drains
- Involvement of apical nodes should be recorded separately

VII.3 Minimal requirements for information from surgeon to pathologist

See also "pathologic examination, tissue sampling and reporting of breast specimens" (Chapter V). If possible, the specimen should be delivered immediately, unfixed and intact to the pathology laboratory. A good communication between surgeon and pathologist is very important to come to an exact diagnosis and treatment plan. Therefore, however time consuming, it is mandatory to provide the pathologist with the following information concerning the breast specimen.

a. Clinical situation of the primary tumor

Exact information on clinical data of the primary tumor is very important.
Please indicate:

- side of the tumor
- clinical size of the tumor
- location of the tumor
- involvement of adjacent tissue
- clinical status of regional lymph nodes

This is done preferably with a schematic drawing and a statement of the clinical TNM status of the primary tumor.

b. Orientation in surgical specimen

For an exact diagnostic work up, the pathologist has to know how the specimen was situated in loco.

For all local excision procedures (excisional biopsy, lumpectomy, segmentectomy, quadrantectomy), the nipple side of the specimen and the basal side (fascia) should be marked (e.g. by long and short sutures).

Together with the provided schematic drawing, the pathologist is then able to locate the lesion in the breast and may be able to indicate possible residual tumor in cases with irradical excisions (e.g. DCIS or EIC positive cases).

Simple mastectomy (ablation) specimen should be marked at the cranial side of the nipple ("12 o'clock" position) and the axillary tail; e.g. by long or short sutures.

In radical mastectomy specimens (and all its modifications) the breast is marked cranially ("12 o'clock"). The en-bloc excised axillary clearance specimen, the apex nodes (level III), the interpectoral nodes and the upper lateral border of the axilla are marked (e.g. with sutures or colored beads).

If node biopsies are performed to guide therapy (apex biopsy, sentinel node biopsy), this should be mentioned and the location of removed nodes should be described in detail.

An axillary dissection specimen is marked at the basis (axillary tail of the breast), at the top (nodes at level II or III) and at the upper-lateral border of the axilla, with sutures or – preferably – with colored beads; the location of the highest axillary nodes on the specimen should be recorded exactly. If top nodes are removed seperately for diagnostic/prognostic purposes, this should be mentioned on the forms, giving details on location.

66

VIII.   Primary treatment: radiotherapy

VIII.1   Introduction

The purpose of this chapter is to establish minimal quality requirements concerning the most relevant issues of curative local and regional irradiation of breast cancer. Standards have to be set to get reliable and comparable data on the treatment results and complications within trials to be performed. Minimal requirements concerning target volumes, treatment standards, dose prescription, treatment delivery and equipment are described and may serve as a guideline to write the radiotherapy chapter of new protocols.

Although many items depend on definitions and specifications that all radiation oncologists agree upon, some issues may be less straightforward. Indications for irradiation of particular regions may change with time and depend upon the protocol that is to be written. For instance, in a trial on partial breast irradiation for low risk patients, it would be absurd to consider whole breast irradiation as a minimum requirement. Similarly, for a study investigating Intensity Modulated Radiotherapy (IMRT) for breast cancer, the mentioned minimum requirements would not be entirely appropriate. The pros and cons of the irradiation of the various regions according to the available evidence in the autumn of 2003 will therefore be briefly discussed as well as the minimum requirements according to current general practice. It is left to the discretion of the protocol writing committee to decide on the indication of irradiation of the particular regions in particular trials, depending upon the questions at stake.

VIII.2 Target volumes

Since local and regional breast irradiation is in many centers not (yet) prepared with a CT based simulation; the typical rules of delineating a Gross Tumour Volume (GTV) with a particular margin to define a Planning Target Volume (PTV) are not entirely applicable here. Yet a description of the GTV or Clinical Target Volume (CTV) is given [1]. Apart from that, field borders will be indicated needed to achieve adequate irradiation of the PTV in case conventional simulation is used.

a. Breast

Whole breast irradiation is indicated after lumpectomy in (standard) breast conservation for early stage breast cancer and DCIS. Furthermore it is indicated in breast conserving treatment of locally advanced breast cancer (LABC) after neo adjuvant chemotherapy and limited surgery and in irresectable LABC.

The CTV for whole breast irradiation is the breast gland. In case of LABC with skin involvement the skin is also part of the CTV or GTV, particularly in case of inflammatory disease.

Organs At Risk (OAR) are the lung and the heart.

The breast is typically irradiated with two tangential beams. With conventional simulation the upper, lower and medial field border should minimally be chosen 1.5 cm superior, inferior and medial of the palpable breast tissue respectively. The lateral field border should be chosen such that the palpable breast tissue in the depth lies well ventrolateral of the projected dorsal match plane of the fields. It is advised to use a technique that creates dorsal match plane alignment (for instance half beam technique) and uses wedge filters or other compensators.

The chance of severe lung toxicity increases if the Central Lung Distance (distance of the inner surface of the ribcage to the dorsal field edge in the center of the simulation film) exceeds 3 cm. Similarly, (late) heart toxicity is possibly increased if the maximum heart distance exceeds 2 cm.

b. Chest wall

Irradiation of the chest wall after Modified Radical Mastectomy (MRM) is indicated in case of large primary tumors (pT3) or more than 3 positive axillary nodes at Axillary Lymph Node Dissection (ALND) because it diminishes local recurrence rate threefold and has an impact on survival. It must be noted that the evidence for this is derived from trials where loco-regional irradiation was used. Furthermore locoregional irradiation is indicated in the multi-modality treatment of LABC or in any other case where the resection margins of the MRM are tumor positive.

The CTV consists of the entire scar of the mastectomy that is, both the deep and superficial dissection plane of the operation. The skin should not be treated to 100% of the dose, except in case of LABC with skin involvement particularly inflammatory disease, or manifest incomplete resection in the skin. OAR: the underlying lung and the heart.

The chest wall can be irradiated with tangential fields like the intact breast, or by electron fields. In the latter case care should be taken to choose the electron energy not too high to avoid irradiation of the lung (and the heart in case of left-sided cancer). Attention should be paid to matching with other fields, for instance by using half beam techniques.

c. Axillary lymph nodes

The indication for axillary irradiation is not entirely clear. The evidence for a survival benefit of postoperative irradiation for intermediate and high-risk patients, shown by the Early Breast Cancer Clinical Trialists Group is based on randomized clinical trials, in which loco regional irradiation was applied, including axillary and medial supraclavicular irradiation. It is however unclear whether the advantage is due to the prevention of local recurrence per se or to the adjuvant regional irradiation. It is advised to consider loco regional irradiation in pN2 disease (more than 3 tumor positive nodes at ALND, and in LABC. Whether axillary irradiation instead of ALND could be used in case of a tumor positive sentinel node is subject to a current EORTC trial (10981/22013 AMAROS).

The CTV consists of the three levels of the axillary lymph nodes and is usually extended to the supraclavicular lymph nodes. Level 1 of the axilla extends from the lateral chest wall in the midaxillary line to the lateral aspect of the minor pectoral muscle. Level 2 lies directly underneath this muscle. Level 3 extends from the medial aspect of the minor pectoral muscle and the costoclavicular ligament. OAR: brachial plexus, shoulder joint, spinal cord.

Typically the axillary region and the supraclavicular region are irradiated with a large AP field, a lateral additional PA field and a medial additional AP field. The large AP field covers the axillary levels and supraclavicular nodes. The lateral additional PA field serves to achieve an adequate dose to the midaxillary region in level 1 and 2. The additional AP field should achieve an adequate dose at 3 cm depth at level 3 and the supraclavicular region. The so-called two fields modified Mc. Whirter techniques (large AP field, additional lateral posterior field) are discouraged because of inhomogeneous dose, particularly in the anterior part of the major pectoral muscle and the brachial plexus. Attention should be paid to matching with tangential breast fields or chest wall fields. It is advisable to use individual blocking of the acromioclavicular joint and lateral part of the humerus. Techniques based upon CT based planning with exact delineation of the CTV and PTV, for instance using Intensity Modulated Radiation Therapy (IMRT) is of course allowed, provided the PTV dose is adequate.

d. Internal Mammary lymph nodes

It is unknown whether or when irradiation of the Internal Mammary Chain (IMC) is indicated. For early disease, this question will be answered after maturation of EORTC trial 22922/10925. The results are expected in 2011. The chance of involved internal mammary lymph nodes increases with tumor load, particularly for patients with medially located tumors. It can be considered in locally advanced disease and in patients with a tumor positive internal mammary sentinel node.

The CTV consists of the ipsilateral internal mammary lymph nodes. OAR: the heart. Often, the IMC nodes are treated together with the supraclavicular nodes that can be considered the upper level/margin of the IMC. These can be considered separately as well. The IMC lymph nodes are located in the first four ipsilateral intercostal spaces, between the dorsal border of the sternum and the pleura. They are difficult to visualize on a CT scan. Lymphoscintigraphy after injection of a radiolabelled tracer in the skin near the xiphoid can indicate the location of the IMC node chain. The vast majority of the IMC nodes fit in an anterior field of 6 cm wide, encompassing the first four intercostal spaces, extending from 1 cm contra lateral of the midline to 5 cm homolateral of the midline, of which the dose should be specified at 3 cm deep. In obese patients with abundant subcutaneous tissue, it may be necessary to specify the dose deeper than 3 cm. This is highly arbitrary, as is the decision on how to deal with overlap of an IMC field with the tangential beams in case both are considered indicated.

e. Supraclavicular lymph nodes

The medial supraclavicular nodes form the upper level of the IMC as well as of the axillary lymph nodes. Supraclavicular recurrences are as common as axillary recurrences. It is recommended to irradiate the supraclavicular nodes whenever axillary or IMC irradiation or both are indicated.

The CTV consists of the supraclavicular nodes. The OAR is the spinal cord. To encompass this in a single anterior field, the medial border should be on the level of the origin of the sterno-cleido-mastoid muscle on the sternum and the caudal border just caudal of the sterno-clavicular joint (see also above).

f. Boost

Boost irradiation is indicated in breast conservation for early stage breast cancer, since it reduces the annual odds of breast relapse by 35–50%. However, the risk of breast relapse after complete excision and whole breast irradiation in women over 60 years is very low. Therefore, the boost treatment may be avoided in this patient group. Furthermore, boost irradiation is indicated in LABC (after lumpectomy or in case of macroscopic residual tumor). Whether boost irradiation is indicated in case of breast conservation for DCIS is unknown.

The CTV for boost irradiation in BCT is the rim of breast tissue surrounding the excision cavity. The optimal margin is arbitrary, as well as the question whether this margin should be larger in case of excision of residual tumor after neo adjuvant chemotherapy for LABC. The GTV for boost irradiation in case of macroscopic tumor is the macroscopic tumor.

Boost doses can be delivered with photons, electrons or with brachytherapy and the choice is arbitrary. The advantage of brachytherapy is irradiation of a smaller volume. With electrons usually a smaller volume is irradiated than with photons. The disadvantage of electrons is a higher chance of (late) skin toxicity.

VIII.3   Treatment standards

Data acquisition and treatment position

Patients are usually treated in supine position with the ipsilateral arm raised aside or above the head and supported. An inclined plane or table wedge may be used and may facilitate optimal sparing of the lung when using matching fields. For planning purposes at least one (preferably more) accurate contour of the patient in the center of the breast should be obtained, preferably with indication of the lung contour. CT simulation is performed in an increasing number of institutions. The difficulty with CT scanners with an aperture of 70 cm is that many patients do not fit in the CT scanner in treatment position, particularly when table wedges are used.

Simulation and dose computation

All fields should be simulated and documented. In case of loco regional treatment, care should be taken to avoid overlap of fields by applying half beam or other matching techniques. Dose distributions should be calculated using adequate 3D treatment planning systems, preferably combining the calculations of all fields.

Dose prescription and specification

The typical dose for breast, chest wall or loco regional irradiation is between 45–50 Gy in 1.8 to 2 Gy fractions, five fractions per week. So far no clinical apparent difference has been proven of other (biologically equivalent) schemes. Boost doses, if indicated are usually between 15 and 25 Gy. It is plausible to consider higher boost doses in case of a higher tumor load, as for instance in irresistible LABC, or in case of incomplete resection.

The dose should be specified according to ICRU standards [1]. That is at the intersection of beam axes in case of opposed or tangential fields. In case the intersection of beam axes is not a relevant point, like in half beam techniques, another, relevant point in the CTV should be appointed. For single photon fields (IMC, infra and supraclavicular area) a relevant point at 3 cm deep should be appointed. For electrons, the dose should always be specified at 100%, and the energy should be chosen such that the depth is adequate.

PTV doses should preferably be kept between 95% and 107% of the prescribed dose. It should be kept above 85% in electron beams (according to ICRU report 52). In order to obtain reliable and comparable data concerning the radiation doses, attention should be paid to clear unambiguous definitions of dose specification points, when writing a multicenter protocol.

Treatment verification

Adequate measures should be taken to achieve a reproducible patient positioning in order to deliver the dose according to the fields as defined and documented during simulation. Each field should be treated every day. At least once, at the beginning of the treatment series a portal image of the treatment fields should be made to verify their correct position.

VIII.4 Minimal quality requirements for protocol prescriptions

Treatment prescriptions

- Clear definition of target volumes, particularly CTV and PTV
- Definition of organs at risk (OAR) and their tolerance levels
- Clear dose prescription, total dose, fraction dose, overall treatment time
- Indication of allowed heterogeneity levels

Treatment preparation

- Define exact treatment position and acceptable variations
- Ensure data acquisition in treatment position
- Suggest simulation techniques to optimize PTV dose and minimize OAR dose
- Prescribe minimum planning requirements to document heterogeneity
- Clearly define ICRU reference points
- Define what doses (e.g. reference, minimum, maximum) should be reported

Treatment delivery

- Prescribe how to ensure reproducibility of treatment.
- Define how to verify accuracy of treatment delivery
- Describe protocol bound quality assurance measures (e.g. Dummy Run)

Outcome measures

- Describe how and when to score early toxicity
- Describe how and when to score late toxicity
- Describe study endpoints adequately

Reference

1. www.icru.org; report 50 and 51.

IX. Adjuvant systemic therapy

IX.1 Introduction

While various nuances of adjuvant systemic therapy are under clinical investigation in the continual search for improvements in survival and care of patients with early breast cancer, it is possible to make several general statements about currently recommended adjuvant therapy.

The recently published updates of the Oxford overview of adjuvant polychemotherapy and hormonal therapy showed convincing reductions in the odds of recurrence and death in practically all groups of early breast cancer patients [1, 2]. Therefore, adjuvant systemic therapy is recommended for all patients with early breast cancer with the following exceptions: adjuvant chemotherapy for patients over the age of 70, due to the paucity of clinical trial data in this group, definitive recommendations are not yet possible; and for patients with minimal-risk disease the decision of whether to treat with adjuvant chemotherapy should depend on the individual risk-benefit analysis.

IX.2   Hormonal therapy

Recommendations for adjuvant hormonal therapy are basically derived from the conclusions of the Oxford overview of hormonal therapy [1,3] and St Gallen consensus on prognostic factors [4].

Tamoxifen

Adjuvant tamoxifen 20 mg/day for five years is recommended for all women with hormone receptor positive breast cancer, regardless of menopausal status, age, or Her-2 status. Whether women with very low risk node negative breast cancer, specifically <1 cm, or 1–2 cm and grade I histology and more than 35 years of age, derive similar benefits from tamoxifen as women with slightly higher risk is not known [4]. Evidence suggests that tamoxifen reduces the risk of contralateral breast cancer, and thus secondary prevention may be a reason to consider tamoxifen in this group of women. For women with tumors that are negative for estrogen and progesterone receptors, the benefit of tamoxifen is debatable. In this scenario, tamoxifen is not recommended.

Anastrozole

The recent results of ATAC trial [5] suggest that anastrozole may be superior to tamoxifen as adjuvant therapy for postmenopausal women. However, no overall survival results are available yet and a longer follow-up is needed to confirm these results. Therefore, 5-years of adjuvant tamoxifen remain the standard therapy and anastrozole should be considered for those postmenopausal patients in whom tamoxifen is contraindicated or not tolerated well.

Further, in a recently published study, the aromatase inhibitor letrozole in addition to five years of adjuvant tamoxifen, show a statistically significant improvement in disease-free survival for the extended adjuvant endocrine treatment (relative risk reduction 43%; absolute gain of 7% for node-positive disease and 3% for node-negative disease). In view of uncertainty regarding long-term risks associated with extended adjuvant letrozole therapy, the decision to offer this therapy after 5 years of tamoxifen needs to be individualized.

Ovarian ablation

Ovarian ablation has been shown to improve survival and reduce breast cancer recurrence in women <50 years old compared with control [3]. For premenopausal women with endocrine-responsive disease ovarian function suppression (goserelin) with [6] or without tamoxifen [7] appeared to be at least as effective as CMF chemotherapy alone, and information is available that the addition of tamoxifen and goserelin is more effective than goserelin alone, at least in the presence of chemotherapy [8]. The sequential use of goserelin after CMF appeared better than either modality alone, at least in women younger than 40 years [9]. Because no firm recommendation can be made on the basis of a subset analysis, the benefit of LHRH agonists in combination with tamoxifen or exemestane will be compared to tamoxifen alone in young women with hormone receptor positive tumors who retain functional ovaries after adjuvant chemotherapy in the context of a Breast International Group (BIG) trial.

When both chemotherapy and hormonal therapy are used, the sequential administration of tamoxifen after completing chemotherapy is recommended. The recent publication of the Intergroup Trial 0100 elegantly showed that sequential administration of tamoxifen and chemotherapy is superior to concurrent use of both modalities [10].

Predictive markers

Estrogen and progesterone receptor content in the primary tumor are the only confirmed markers that predict responsiveness to hormonal therapy in breast cancer. Data on the predictive value of Her-2 overexpression for response to hormonal therapy and anthracycline containing chemotherapy is inconsistent. Therefore, the predictive utility of Her-2 overexpression awaits confirmation.

Ongoing investigations

Currently active randomized controlled trials of adjuvant hormone therapy are examining whether more than 5 years of tamoxifen is superior to 5 years; whether aromatase inhibitors or new selective estrogen receptor modulators really provide similar or superior risk reduction with fewer side effects (particularly less endometrial proliferation and lower risk of thromboembolic disease); whether sequential tamoxifen and aromatase inhibitors enhance survival compared with tamoxifen alone; and the role of ovarian ablation plus tamoxifen or aromatase inhibitors in the treatment of premenopausal women who do not receive chemotherapy or remain premenopausal after chemotherapy. Preliminary answers to these research questions should be available in the next few years.

IX.3 Chemotherapy

Recommendations for adjuvant chemotherapy are derived from conclusions of the Oxford overview of polychemotherapy [2] and St Gallen consensus on prognostic factors [4].

When to give chemotherapy

The Oxford overview showed that the treatment with adjuvant chemotherapy is associated with highly significant absolute reductions in death for premenopausal node negative (7%) and node positive (11%) breast cancer, and postmenopausal node negative (2%) and node positive (3%) breast cancer, regardless of the simultaneous use of tamoxifen [2]. Therefore, chemotherapy is recommended for all women with estrogen and progesterone receptor negative tumors, even when other prognostic factors are favorable. For women with hormone receptor positive tumors, chemotherapy is recommended for lymph node-positive patients and for the patients with larger tumors, lymphatic or vascular tumor emboli, high histological grade and for younger patients, regardless the lymph node status. For those with lymph node-negative disease the use of chemotherapy in addition to hormonal therapy should be based on balancing the absolute risk reductions with expected side effects of the treatment. According to the recently published results, hormonal therapy alone may be adequate adjuvant therapy for node negative postmenopausal disease [11, 12] as well as for premenopausal endocrine responsive disease [6, 7, 13]. However, for any firm conclusions confirmatory studies are needed. On the other hand, chemotherapy alone is insufficient treatment for younger patients with hormone receptor positive disease. In a retrospective analysis, conducted in parallel across multiple cooperative groups, chemotherapy alone was found to be associated with inadequate survival benefit in younger patients [14].

What chemotherapy to give

The choice of chemotherapy regimen depends on recurrence risk, co-morbid illness and patient preference. In the Oxford overview anthracycline based chemotherapy was found to be associated with a 12% reduction in the annual odds of recurrence and an 11% reduction in the annual odds of death compared with CMF, however toxicity, especially cardiac, was slightly higher [2]. Anthracycline based chemotherapy should be considered for women with high risk disease and CMF for women with either modest relapse risk or contraindications to anthracycline therapy. According to the retrospective findings, across several clinical trials [15, 16], anthracycline-containing regimens may be superior to non-anthracycline–containing regimens in Her-2 positive disease. Dose intensification of anthracyclines and cyclophos-phamide have thus far failed to show an advantage over conventional regimens, such as AC 60/600 mg/m^2 or regimens containing epirubicin 75–90 mg/m^2 [17, 18], however suboptimal dose-intensity and/or cumulative doses are clearly linked with inferior survival [17, 19, 20]. High dose chemotherapy with stem cell transplant after induction chemotherapy has not been shown to enhance survival or significantly reduce recurrence in several trials [21–24]. Another concept recently examined in a large randomized trial is that of dose density. In contrast to a few negative trials, the recently published trial comparing 2-week dose dense schedule with the growth factors support to a 3-week schedule confirmed the superiority of dose density schedule in terms of disease-free and overall survival [25]. However, for any firm conclusions on the value of dose-dense chemotherapy regimens in breast cancer patients at last one large confirmatory trial is desirable and every effort should be made to identify the subset of women, which derives a large benefit from this approach.

Taxanes

There is suggestion that the addition of a taxane in the adjuvant regimen may enhance survival in node positive breast cancer [26, 27]. However, there is substantial concern with the choice of the "control arm" in these trials. Further follow-up of these studies and other confirmatory studies with stronger control arms are required before definitive conclusions, on the value of taxanes in the adjuvant setting, are to be made. Numerous trials with more than 20,000 women included are to be reported in a few years. The use of a taxane in the adjuvant setting outside a clinical trial cannot currently be recommended.

Predictive markers

So far there are no confirmed predictive markers for response to chemotherapy. The predictive utility of Her-2 overexpression, cell proliferation markers and some other markers are under investigation and await confirmation. Although overexpression of Her-2 is associated with increased risk of breast cancer relapse and more aggressive disease, its predictive value in response to chemotherapy is not yet well understood [28]. According to the data available [15, 16], preference for anthracyclines over CMF may be reasonable for women with Her-2 overexpressing tumors. However, confirmatory prospective data is required. On the other hand the predictive value of Her-2 overexpression for response to trastuzumab has been confirmed in the metastatic setting. Investigations of adjuvant trastuzumab for patients with Her-2 overexpressing tumors are underway and its use outside of clinical trials is currently not justified.

Ongoing questions

Several different adjuvant chemotherapy strategies are under investigation, including incorporation of taxanes either sequentially or concurrently to anthracyclines; exploration of the added value of trastuzumab in Her-2 overexpressing tumors; investigation of dose-dense schedules and comparing the combination of chemotherapy with ovarian ablation ($+/-$ tamoxifen or aromatase inhibitors) to either modality alone in premenopausal women.

IX.4 Preoperative systemic therapy

Preoperative systemic therapy, also known as up-front, induction or neoadjuvant therapy is given before the standard loco-regional therapy (before surgery and/or radiotherapy). Not only it might have an effect on potential micrometastases (survival) but also has an effect on the local regional tumor growth (with hence a possible indirect effect on survival).

For inoperable locally advanced disease, the initial use of anthracycline-based preoperative chemotherapy is standard management. Local therapy after preoperative therapy usually consists of surgery, which can even be conservative, and irradiation of chest wall (breast) and supraclavicular nodes, followed by hormonal treatment if the tumor is hormonal receptive positive.

Preoperative systemic therapy, especially chemotherapy, increases the rate of breast-conserving surgery in women presenting with large, unifocal operable breast cancer [29]. In schedules using anthracyclines alone or anthracycline-taxane combinations high pathological complete response rates as well as high rates of breast conserving surgery can be achieved [29]. The superiority of preoperative chemotherapy over adjuvant (postoperative) chemotherapy in terms of overall survival has not been demonstrated. It could be used in selected patients presenting with unifocal tumors, too large for immediate breast conserving surgery, if the patient prefers breast conservation after being informed about the risks and benefits of preoperative chemotherapy. After the preoperative treatment the patient should have a repeat mammography and be carefully evaluated to decide if breast conversion became feasible. Response registration should not only include survival data and toxicity but also the effect on the local regional tumor growth (see X.1).

In elderly patients a substantial rate of tumor reduction can be achieved with hormonal therapy using tamoxifen [30]. New generation of aromatase inhibitors also proved to be highly effective in achieving clinical responses rates and breast conservation rates in postmenopausal women with endocrine-responsive disease [31]. However, due to the lack of data on long-term local control as well as on survival, preoperative hormonal therapy cannot yet be recommended for treatment out of clinical trials, except for elderly and frail patients with large ER/PgR positive tumors.

References

1. Early Breast Cancer Trialists Collaborative Group. Tamoxifen for early breast cancer: an overview of the randomised trials. *Lancet* 351:1451–1467, 1998
2. Early Breast Cancer Trialists Collaborative Group. Polychemotherapy for early breast cancer: an overview of the randomised trials. *Lancet* 352:930–942, 1998
3. Early Breast Cancer Trialists' Collaborative Group. Ovarian ablation in early breast cancer: overview of the randomised trials. *Lancet* 348:1189–1196, 1996
4. Goldhirsch A, Wood WC, Gelber RD, Coates AS, Thurlimann B, Senn HJ. Meeting highlights: Updated international expert consensus panel on the primary therapy of early breast cancer. *J Clin Oncol* 21:1–9, 2003
5. The ATAC Trialists' Group. Anastrozole alone or in combination with tamoxifen versus tamoxifen alone for adjuvant treatment of postmenopausal women with early breast cancer: first results of the ATAC randomised trial. *Lancet* 2002; 359:2131–2139

6. Jakesz R, Hausmaninger H, Kubista E, et al. Randomized adjuvant trial of tamoxifen and goserelin versus cyclophosphamide, methotrexate and fluorouracil: Evidence for the superiority of treatment with endocrine blockade in premenopausal patients with hormone responsive breast cancer – Austrian Breast and Colorectal Cancer Study Group Trial 5. *J Clin Oncol* 20:4621–4627, 2002

7. Jonat V, Kaufmann M, Sauerbrei W, et al. Goserelin versus cyclophosphamide, methotrexate and fluorouracil as adjuvant therapy in premenopausal patients with node-positive breast cancer: The Zoladex Early Breast Cancer Research Association Study. *J Clin Oncol* 20:4628–4635, 2002

8. Davidson N, O'Neill A, Vukov A, et al. Effect of chemohormonal therapy in premenopausal, node positive, receptor positive breast cancer: An Eastern Cooperative Oncology Group phase III Intergroup trial. *Proc Am Soc Clin Oncol* 18:67a, 1999 (abstract 249)

9. Castiglione – Gertsch M, O'Neill A, Gelber RD, et al. Is the addition of adjuvant chemotherapy always neccesary in node negative (N−) pre/perimenopausal breast cancer patients who receive goserelin? First results of IBCSG trial VIII. *Proc Am Soc Clin Oncol* 21:38a, 2002 (abstract 149)

10. Albain KS, Green SJ, Ravdin PM, et al. Adjuvant chemohormonal therapy for primary breast cancer should be sequential instead of concurrent: initial results from Intergroup trial 0100 (SWOG-8814). *Proc Am Soc Clin Oncol* 21:37a, 2002 (abstract 143)

11. Fisher B, Jeong J-H, Bryant J, et al. Findings from two decades of National Surgical Adjuvant Breast and Bowel Project clinical trials involving breast cancer with negative axillary nodes. Proceedings of San Antonio Breast Cancer Symposium, December 11–14, 2002, san Antonio, TX (abstract 16)

12. International Breast Cancer Study Group. Endocrine responsiveness and tailoring adjuvant therapy for postmenopausal lymph node-negative breast cancer: A randomized trial. *J Natl Cancer Inst* 94:1054–1065, 2002

13. International Breast Cancer Study Group. Randomized controlled trial of ovarian function suppression plus tamoxifen versus the same endocrine therapy plus chemotherapy: is chemotherapy necessary for premenopausal women with node-positive breast cancer? First results of International Breast Cancer Study Group Trail 11–93. *Breast* 10:130–138, 2001 (suppl 3)

14. Goldhirsch A, Gelber RD, Yothers G, et al. Adjuvant therapy for very young women with breast cancer: Need for tailored treatments. *J Natl Cancer Inst Monogr* 30:44–51, 2001

15. Paik S, Bryant J, Park C, et al. ErbB-2 and response to doxorubicin in patients with axillary lymph node-positive hormone receptor – negative breast cancer. *J Natl Cancer Inst* 90:1361–1370, 1998

16. Thor AD, Berry DA, Budman DR. ErbB-2, p53, and efficacy of adjuvant therapy in lymph node-positive breast cancer. *J Natl Cancer Inst* 90:1346–1360, 1998

17. Wood WC, Budman DR, Korzun AH, et al. Dose and dose intensity of adjuvant chemotherapy for stage II, node-positive breast carcinoma. *N Engl J Med* 330:1253–1259, 1994

18. Fisher B, Anderson S, Wickerham DL, et al. Increased intensification and total dose of cyclophosphamide in a doxorubicin-cyclophosphamide regimen for the treatment of primary breast cancer: findings from National Surgical Adjuvant Breast and Bowel Project B-22. *J Clin Oncol* 15:1858–1869, 1997

19. Engelsman E, Klijn JCM, Rubens RD, et al. "Classical" CMF versus a 3-weekly intravenous CMF schedule in postmenopausal patients with advanced breast cancer. An EORT Breast Cancer Co-operative Group Phase III Trial (10808). *Eur J Cancer* 27:966–970, 1991

20. Biganzoli L, Piccart MJ. The bigger the better? ... or what we know and what we still need to learn about anthracycline dose per course, dose density and cumulative dose in the treatment of breast cancer [editorial] *Ann Oncol* 8:1177–1182, 1997

21. Peters W, Rosner G, Vredenburgh J, et al. A prospective, randomized comparison of two doses of combination alkylating agents as consolidation after AC in high-risk primary breast cancer involving ten or more axillary lymph nodes: Preliminary Results of CALGB 9082/SWOG 9114/NCIC MA-13. *Proc Am Soc Clin Oncol* 18:1a, 1999 (abstract)

22. The Scandinavian Breast Cancer Study Group 9401. Results from a randomized adjuvant breast cancer study with high dose chemotherapy with CTCb supported by autologous bone marrow stem cells versus dose escalated and tailored FEC therapy. *Proc Am Soc Clin Oncol* 18:2a, 1999 (abstract)

23. Rodenhuis S, Richel DJ, van der Wall E, et al. Randomised trial of high-dose chemotherapy and haemopoietic progenitor-cell support in operable breast cancer with extensive axillary lymph-node involvement. *The Lancet* 352:515–521, 1998

24. Hortobagyi GN, Buzdar AU, Theriault RL, et al. Randomized trial of high-dose chemotherapy and blood cell autografts for high-risk primary breast carcinoma. *J Natl Cancer Inst* 92:225–233, 2000

25. Citron MI, Berry DA, Cirrincione C, et al. Randomized trial of dose-dense versus conventionally scheduled and sequential versus concurrent combination chemotherapy

26. Henderson IC, Berry DA, Demetri G, et al. Improved outcomes from adding sequential paclitaxel but not from escalating doxorubicin dose in an adjuvant chemotherapy regimen for patients with node-positive primary breast cancer. *J Clin Oncol* 21:1–9, 2003 (abstract 390A)

27. Nabholtz J-M, Pienkowski T, Mackey J, et al. Phase III trial comparing TAC (docetaxel, doxorubicin, cyclophosphamide) with FAC (5-fluorouracil, doxorubicin, cyclophosphamide) in the adjuvant treatment of node positive breast cancer (BC) patients: interim analysis of the BCIRG 001 study. *Proc Am Soc Clin Oncol* 21:36a, 2002 (abstract 141)

28. Piccart MJ, Di Leo A, and Hamilton A. HER2: A "predictive factor" ready to use in daily management of breast cancer patients? *Eur J Cancer* 36:1755–1761, 2000

29. Wolmark N, Wang J, Mamounas E, Bryant J, Fisher B. Preoperative chemotherapy in patients with operable breast cancer: nine-year results from national Surgical adjuvant Breast and Bowel Project B-18. *J Natl cancer Inst Monogr* 30:96–102, 2001

30. Mustacchi G, Latteier J, Baum M, et al. Tamoxifen alone vs. surgery plus tamoxifen for breast cancer of the elderly: Meta-analysis of long-term results of the GRETA and CRC trials. *Breast Cancer Res Treat* 50:227–346, 1998

31. Ellis MJ, Coop A, Singh B, et al. Letrozole is more effective neoadjuvant endocrine therapy than tamoxifen for ErbB-1- and/or ErbB-2-positive, estrogen receptor-positive primary breast cancer: Evidence from a phase III randomized trial. *J Clin Oncol* 19:3808–3816, 2001

X. Primary treatment evaluation

X.1   Requirements for evaluation of treatment results

X.2   Cosmesis

X.3   Functional sequelae

X.4   Follow-up schedules after treatment of primary breast cancer with curative intent

X.5   Recording first recurrence and calculating disease-free interval

X.1 Requirements for evaluation of treatment results

Pathologic reports should be complete and reliable with regard to margin evaluation, tumor type, size of the tumor, presence of an intraductal component, axillary lymph node status, receptor status and other prognostic markers. The original site of the tumor should be registered according to the definitions in IV.1 and the site of a recurrence should be registered according to the same system. All local recurrences should be confirmed by histology or cytology (FNAC). A baseline mammography (postoperative/pre-radiotherapy) is advisable to rule out residual suspect microcalcifications and to have a reference for future follow-up mammographies. The extent of surgery should be documented in detail from the beginning, especially with regard to the extend of the axillary clearance. Details on sentinel node procedure should be included. Radiotherapy reports should include dose, fractionation schedule, used energy, fields and duration of the treatment. Brachytherapy modalities should be documented in the same way. Follow-up and cosmetic evaluation should be uniform and well documented with respect to all essential items. In patients with local recurrences after breast conserving therapy, details on salvage treatment and treatment results should be available. The administration of adjuvant systemic therapy should be specified with regard to type, dose, type of administration and time schedule. The effect of upfront systemictherapy (neoadjuvant therapy) should include the local regional response. Apart from careful clinical measurements of the treatment response, mammographic (and/or US and/or MRI) evaluation, compared to the pre-treatment evaluations is mandatory. CT scan and PET scan might give additional information. Complete remission can only by stated if at careful pathology investigation of the loco-regional tumor site no tumor has been found. (Pathological complete remission). If no pathology confirmation is possible or available, it should always be stated that the response was evaluated on clinical bases.

X.2 Cosmesis

Cosmetic assessment following breast conserving therapy is important since a good cosmetic result is one of the two major end points (apart from the local control) in this therapy modality. Surgical sequelae may lead to breast asymmetry due to volume loss or contour deformation. Radiotherapy, depending on dose, volume and fractionation, may aggravate asymmetry and deformation by increasing breast fibrosis, or may course skin damage such as pigmentation, depigmentation of the areola and on the long term visible skin teleangiectasia. Chemotherapy may enhance the effects of radiation and increase the incidence of fibrosis, teleangiectasia and pigmentation.

For qualitative evaluation of cosmesis a four-point scale should be used: excellent (no visible sequelae), good (visible, but not disturbing sequelae), fair (marked sequelae), poor (unacceptable sequelae). A panel should preferably perform qualitative evaluation of cosmesis. The number of panel members should be at least 5 and the group should include lay people and female persons. Hereby, the risk of underscoring or overscoring will be minimized. The panel member should be shown and should discuss examples of the different categories to lessen the interobserver variability. Total results and more detailed items can be studied, depending on type of treatment and trial purpose. For the data interpretation, sometimes a dichotomization of the categories (excellent/good versus fair/poor) is acceptable. It is advised that photographs are taken, with the consent of the patient, after surgery, before radiotherapy, and every three years thereafter. Each time three pictures should be taken with the patient standing. Two frontal views from neck to abdomen, one with arms raised, one with arms alongside the body and one profile view (taken from the treatment side) with arms raised. On the frontal picture with the patient having arms alongside, trunk marks on the skin should be made at the incisura jugularis (+) and at the midline 25 cm lower (+) to allow calculation of the correction magnification factor (this is necessary for the quantitative assessment). In any analysis of the cosmetic result, the length of follow-up should be carefully considered and if possible changes over time should be studied.

Quantitative assessment of asymmetry of breast contour and nipple position. The following measurements will be made on the photograph and can be easily carried out by using the digitizer of a treatment planning system.

On the ordinate: distance A from the incisura jugularis to the nipple level
distance I from the incisura jugularis to the projection of the inferior breast contour.
On the abscissa: distance M from the midline to the nipple
distance L from the midline to the projection of the lateral breast contour.

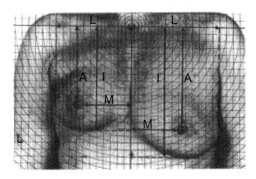

Figure: Scoring system for measurement of breast contour and nipple asymmetries [1].

The distances A, I, M, L shall be measured in the treated breast whereas the distances A′, I′, M′, L′ of the untreated breast will serve as references.

Differences (A′ − A) and (I′ − I) quantify upside retraction of the nipple position and the inferior breast contour, whereas (M′ − M) and (L′ − L) measure asymmetry in the medio-lateral sense. Also differences in the oblique distances between the incisura jugularis and the nipples can be measured as is done by the Breast Retraction Assessment (BRA). This BRA is calculated as follows: [1,2] $(A′ − A)^2 + (M′ − M)$ [2].

For calibration the incisure jugularis and a point at the midline 25 cm lower should be marked on the skin.

Skin damage such as teleangiectasia can be scored by using a modification of the quantitative scale introduced by Turesson [2].

Grade 0: no visible teleangiectasis
Grade 1: less than $2/cm^2$
Grade 2: between $2–4/cm^2$
Grade 3: more than $4/cm^2$
Grade 4: skin necrosis

X.3　Functional sequelae

Surgery and radiotherapy can induce sequelae. Some occur early, others late or even very late. The first evaluation must be done 3 to 4 months after the end of loco-regional treatment, then at the yearly follow-up. Items to evaluate:

Skin – soft tissue – bone

– inflammation, fibrosis, retraction of breast and/or nipple, teleangiectasis, necrosis
– Skin colour changes
– pain in breast (none – little – moderate – severe)
– paralysis of mm latissimus dorsi, pectoralis major, serratus anterior
– rib fractures.

Mobility of the arm (in grades)

– abduction/elevation
– rotation outwards – inwards
– retroflexion.

Edema of the arm

– aspect:　white and soft, firm, tense, fibrosis, inflammatory episodes
– measurements:　circumference forearm and upper arm (at fixed distances (10 cm) above and below olecranon) or by excess volume measurements.

Neuropathy of the plexus brachialis

– mild discomfort in the shoulder
– paresthesia
– weakness in the arm and hand
– pain
– paralysis.

Heart and lung injuries

– pericarditis
– myocardial infarction
– pneumonitis
– fibrosis of the lung.

The quantification of such items is indicated in protocols studying morbidity and side effects (see also X.2 and XIV).

X.4 Follow-up schedules after treatment of primary breast cancer with curative intent

The follow-up starts after the completion of surgery, radiotherapy and/or adjuvant chemotherapy. Routine adjuvant hormonal treatment requires no additional follow-up investigations.

Minimal time schedule

- During the first 2 years: twice a year
- After the first 2 years: annual follow-up visits for life.

Minimal follow-up investigations

- Postoperative mammogram in breast conservation for DCIS detected by microcalcifications
- history
- physical examination with emphasis on the treated site or breast, the contralateral breast and their regional lymph node areas
- general physical examination
- annual mammography/US to be compared with previous mammogram
- all other investigations need only be performed when indicated by history or physical examination.

X.5 Recording first recurrence and calculating disease-free interval

The term recurrence includes all or any of the following:

1. progressive residual disease after local therapy
2. new disease in any area previously treated locally
3. detection of disease outside the locally treated area(s).

Three aspects of recording have to be considered.

Diagnosis of recurrence

One or more of the following must be positive for a diagnosis of tumor recurrence to be accepted, even if symptoms have necessitated a change in management.

- Histology or cytology. Histological proof should be sought at the first appearance of all readily accessible disease. When superficial nodes, a contralateral breast lesion or a fluid collection occur in isolation, histological or cytological proof of diagnosis is regarded as essential.
- Progression of a previously suspicious lesion on the basis of worsening physical signs and/or the detection of tumor not previously shown by imaging tests (e.g. radiographs and scans).
- Objective response (as determined by serial measurements, radiology or photography) of a lesion to specific systemic therapy or local radiotherapy, or
- Autopsy examination.

Any other laboratory test must be supported by one of the above and cannot be taken in isolation either for the diagnosis or the dating of relapse, e.g. abnormal liver function tests or elevated serum calcium or CA 15.3.

Classification of recurrence

Once a suspicious sign is confirmed as due to recurrent cancer, the site of involvement is classified as local, regional, contralateral or distant.

a. Local recurrence

This includes recurrence after mastectomy in the skin or soft tissue of the chest wall within the anatomical area bounded by the mid-sternal line, the clavicle, the posterior axillary line and the costal margin or any type of breast carcinoma in the breast after conservation therapy. Disease occurring in the conserved breast distant from the original primary tumor site (i.e. in a different quadrant) should be separately coded but left within the local category, regardless of initial therapy.

b. Regional disease

This category is for tumor that recurs in lymph nodes draining the primary site namely nodes in the ipsilateral axilla, infraclavicular fossa, and/or lymph nodes in one or both internal mammary chains.

c. Contralateral disease

Only when a discrete contralateral lesion is non-invasive, is invasive with an in-situ component or is of a different histological type than the original breast tumor, is it without doubt a new primary lesion. Involvement of the contralateral breast without any of these features is counted by some as distant spread regardless of the time interval from initial therapy or the time interval from subsequent recurrent disease.

However, subsequent behavior following local therapy may suggest that some of these other lesions also are new primary tumors. Separate classification of all contralateral breast tumors is advocated irrespective of the timing, the way in which they present or are managed. Contralateral axillary or infraclavicular node involvement occurring in conjunction with tumor in the contralateral breast is included in this category, but not contralateral breast involvement contiguous with soft-tissue recurrence in the ipsilateral breast or chest wall (i.e. distant soft tissue spread).

d. Distant spread

All other disease sites are included under this heading and are classified as

- the soft-tissue category
- the visceral category
- skeletal spread.

Time to recurrence

This is based on the detection of a site and never on the onset of a symptom. For consistency and, therefore, comparability of treatment groups within a trial, the date of onset is the date on which a decision is taken by the clinician to investigate a sign. The "date" for a clinically suspicious lesion is the date on which its presence is first recorded in the notes provided action is taken as a result of which the diagnosis is confirmed. The "action date" only becomes the "date of onset" if the action taken confirms (by histology, by further progression or by temporary control following specific tumor therapy) that the suspicion of relapse was founded. Thus confirmation is essential but the *date* of confirmation is irrelevant.

This use of "date of action" reduces variations due to waiting for or agreeing to biopsy and improves comparability of recording within individual trials. For lesions requiring confirmation by imaging techniques, the date of onset is determined in the same way. However, the date may be determined retrospectively following review of previous investigations undertaken before the date of first clinical suspicion. When this is the case, the date of recurrence is the date on which the original investigation was done. Should this back-dating lead to a diagnosis of metastatic disease which precedes initial therapy or trial entry, the date of recurrence is adjusted to give a disease-free interval of zero.

Calculating disease-free interval – disease-free survival

General remark
- Disease-free interval (DFI): for *individual* patients, the disease-free interval can only be assessed if this patient has a local/regional relapse or metastasis and is defined as the *actual* period between the diagnosis of the primary disease and the detection of the first relapse. The length of this period is more or less correlated with the growth velocity of the metastasis. If a patient has already advanced disease at the time of the primary diagnosis or locally advanced disease without a complete clinical response after primary therapy, the disease-free interval is 0 months and has no predictive value with respect to tumor kinetics.

- Disease-free survival (DFS); relapse-free survival (RFS): The disease-free period has a different role in the analyses of primary treatment and metastatic disease. If the "disease-free interval" is used for the analysis of results of therapy in patients with primary breast cancer, it is advised to use the terms disease-free survival or relapse-free survival. In general, these terms are used as expressions for the estimated actuarial percentage of a *group* of patients who are free of disease at a given date after a defined starting point (i.e. diagnosis, primary therapy, randomization, etc.). The date from which it is calculated varies according to the initial therapy [Table 1].

Table 1: Rules for identifying the starting date of the disease-free survival according to disease type and initial therapy.

Disease type	Type of initial therapy	Start of disease-free survival
Operable	Randomized	Date of randomization
	Non-random	Date of excision of tumor
Inoperable	Randomized	Date of randomization
	Non-random irradiation only	Date of end of course giving complete clinical response
	Non-random systemic (+/− XRT)	Date of complete clinical response

For statistical purposes for patients randomized in trials of initial therapy the starting date is the date of randomization while for other surgically treated patients it is the date of tumor excision. In the non-random situation, for patients treated *without* excision of the primary tumor there has to be a complete clinical remission to therapy. For them the DFS starts from the date of completion of radiotherapy or, when systemic therapy has been given, the date when the complete clinical remission is first recorded.

With the introduction of neoadjuvant (upfront) therapy (before surgery and/or radiotherapy) the definition of the starting date for the calculation of the disease-free survival is more complex: in cases with pathology confirmation of complete remission, the date of the clinical complete response should be used. In radically operated cases with still tumor in the specimen present, the date of the operation should be used. In non-operated but exclusively irradiated cases the date of the end of the course giving a complete clinical response should be used.

Once the starting date and the date and site of first relapse are established, the DFS and/or the distant-DFS is calculated. In some protocols, local relapse is not counted as the first failure but merely as an indication for further local therapy, so does not feature in the calculation of the DFS. Similarly, whether to include the development of a second primary breast cancer in the calculation of the DFS for primary therapy trials will depend on the individual protocol. In these trials the subsequent cancer of the other breast may be dealt with separately and not counted as a recurrence.

References

1. Van Limbergen E, van der Schueren E, Vantongelen K. Cosmetic evaluation of breast conserving treatment of mammary cancer. 1. Proposal of a quantitative scoring system. *Radiotherapy and Oncology*, 16: 159–167, 1989.
2. Turesson I, Notter G, The influence of fraction size in radiotherapy on the late normal tissue reaction (I + II). *Int. J. Radiat. Oncol. Biol. Phys.*, 10: 593–606, 1984.
3. Pezner RD, Patterson MD, Hiller HR, Vora N, Desai KR, Aschambeau JO, Lipsett JA. Breast retraction assessment: an objective evaluation of cosmetic results of patients treated conservatively for breast cancer. *Int. J. Radiat. Oncol. Biol. Phys.*, 11, 575–578, 1985.

XI.   Metastatic disease

XI.1 Dominant site of disease

Sites of disease are defined according to the UICC classification.

(i)   The soft-tissue category of distant spread includes:
    (a)   widespread subcutaneous nodules
    (b)   contiguous soft-tissue spread outside the area defined
    (c)   contralateral supraclavicular or cervical lymph nodes of either side
    (d)   contralateral axillary or infraclavicular lymph node involvement with a normal contralateral breast.

(ii)   Skeletal spread, confirmed radiologically, or by the presence of multiple hot spots or by significant changes in sequential bone scans which cannot be explained on radiological examination, is a category on its own.

(iii)   The visceral category is principally for focal deposits in lung, liver or brain but also includes other life-threatening disease such as histologically proven pleural effusions, lymphangitis carcinomatosa of the lung, mediastinal, hilar or intra-abdominal (lymph node) involvement and peritoneal deposits with or without ascites.

Bone marrow involvement, with or without a leukoerythroblastic blood picture, is frequently but not always associated with radiological evidence of skeletal spread and has life-threatening implications similar to those of visceral disease. In contrast, patients with skeletal disease alone may live for many years. Thus, marrow involvement is coded "visceral".

When disease involves more than one category, the patient is classified by the category associated with the worst prognosis irrespective of the extent of involvement. This is the *dominant* site of disease. The order of increasing gravity of prognosis is i, ii, iii. Some protocols may separate single visceral from the category of multiple visceral involvement or even have separate categories for the four different sites of lung, liver, brain and other.

Data forms for new protocols should have a simple table in which tumor load for each category can be recorded. Each protocol should describe the investigations necessary to identify "detectable" disease.

XI.2 Guidelines for investigation of patients for metastatic disease

The pretreatment staging work-up of patients with histologically or cytologically confirmed breast cancer presenting with metastatic disease should include a complete medical history, physical examination, blood tests (hematology with complete blood count; biochemistry, including electrolytes, calcium, albumine, liver function tests, alkaline phosphatase and creatinine; measurements of tumor marker(s) i.e. CA 15.3, chest X-ray, abdominal ultrasound (US)/CT scan, and bone scan. Areas of increased uptake on bone scan should be evaluated with skeletal X-rays and/or CT/MRI to determine whether these represent metastatic disease. Brain MRI or CT should be considered an optional test, but should always be performed in patients presenting with neurologic symptoms. A MRI of the vertebral column should be performed if the neurological signs and symptoms may be compatible with peripheral nervous system involvement. In patients presenting with impaired hematology tests, staging work-up should include bone marrow aspiration and biopsy.

CT scan of the chest is recommended in case of mediastinal and hilar involvement. CT scan of the chest is required for lung lesions not completely surrounded by aerated area on chest X-ray (Response Evaluation Criteria in Solid Tumors – RECIST guidelines). CT scan of the abdomen is required if abnormalities are seen on abdominal US which will be used as target lesions [1].

Cytological or histological confirmation of doubtful lesions as well as of a solitary lesion (RECIST guidelines [1]) is recommended. Estrogen and progesterone receptor analysis as well as Her-2 determination should be performed on any surgical specimen where there is sufficient tissue for both pathologic and tumor markers study.

XI.3 Measurability of tumor lesions at baseline

The lesions which will be used for evaluation of response (target lesions) must be clearly defined at the entry of the patient into the trial.

XI.3.1 Definition of measurable/non-measurable lesions

World Health Organization (WHO) criteria

a. Measurable, bi-dimensional
Malignant disease that can be precisely measured (metric system) in two dimensions by ruler or calipers with surface area determined by multiplying the greatest diameter by the perpendicular diameter. In case of multiple lesions, the total tumor size is defined as the sum of the products of the largest perpendicular diameters of each lesion.

b. Measurable, uni-dimensional
Malignant disease that can be precisely measured (metric system) in one dimension by ruler or calipers.

c. Non-measurable, evaluable
Malignant disease evident on clinical examination but not measurable precisely by ruler or calipers. Lymphangitic or confluent multi-nodular lung metastases, miliary disease on serosal surfaces with or without effusions or meningeal carcinomatosis are all examples of involvement that is evaluable rather than measurable. When applicable, photographs should be taken before and during therapy to document response (e.g. inflammatory cancer).

RECIST criteria

a. Measurable lesions
Lesions that can be accurately measured (metric system) by ruler or calipers in at least one dimension with longest diameter ⩾20 mm. With spiral CT scan, lesions must be ⩾10 mm in at least one dimension.

b. Non-measurable lesions
All other lesions, including small lesions (longest diameter <20 mm with conventional techniques or <10 mm with spiral CT scan) and other non-measurable lesions. These include: bone lesions; leptomeningeal disease; ascite; pleural/pericardial effusion; inflammatory breast disease; lymphangitis cutis/polmonis; abdominal masses that are not confirmed and followed by imaging techniques; and cystic lesions.

XI.3.2 Time of measuring the target lesions

The baseline measurements should be taken just before the start of therapy (<4 weeks before the beginning of treatment according to RECIST [1]). Utilizing baseline measurements that reflect tumor status weeks prior to treatment may well result in an underestimating of treatment effect. The duration of response clearly depends on the frequency and completeness with which the tests are performed: it is therefore essential that diagnostic tests and follow-up intervals for assessing response are precisely specified in the protocol.

XI.3.3 Method of measuring

Objective response can be determined clinically, radiographically, biochemically or by surgicopathologic restaging. The method of determining response should therefore always be specified and the same technique should be used to characterize each identified and reported lesion at baseline and during follow-up. Relevant chemical values and biologic markers should be measured during therapy but cannot be used to evaluate response, unless specifically stipulated in individual protocols.

Specific recommendations from the RECIST guidelines are:

- Clinically detected lesions will only be considered measurable when they are superficial (e.g. skin nodules, palpable lymph nodes). For the case of skin lesions, documentation by color photography – including a ruler to estimate the size of the lesion, is recommended.
- US should not be used to measure tumor lesions that are clinically not easily accessible. It may be used as a possible alternative to clinical measurements of superficial palpable nodes, subcutaneous lesions and thyroid nodules. US might also be useful to confirm the complete disappearance of superficial lesions usually assessed by clinical examination.
- Tumor markers alone cannot be used to assess response. However, if markers are initially above the upper normal limit, they must return to normal levels for a patient to be considered in complete clinical response when all tumor lesions have disappeared.

XI.4 Definitions of objective response

Objective response can be determined clinically, radiographically, biochemically or by surgicopathologic restaging. The method of determining response should therefore always be specified.

WHO criteria

Measurable disease

a. Complete response (CR)
The disappearance of all known disease, determined by 2 observations not less than 4 weeks apart.

b. Partial response (PR)
50% or more decrease in total tumor size of the lesions which have been measured to determine the effect of therapy by 2 observations not less than 4 weeks apart. In addition, there can be no appearance of new lesions or progression of any lesion.

c. Progressive disease (PD)
A 25% or more increase in the size of one or more measurable lesions larger than a specific size, depending the site of the lesion (this should be specified in the protocol (e.g. 10 mm skin lesion and lymph node lesions; 20 mm liver lesions)), or the appearance of new lesions.

d. No change (NC)
A 50% decrease in total tumor size cannot be established nor has a 25% increase in the size of one or more measurable lesions been demonstrated. This is not a category of objective response but if toxicity allows, it is useful as a guide to continue the treatment until either progression or partial response is observed.

N.B. "stabilizations" lasting more than 6 months are often recorded apart and considered in association with partial and complete responses to define the clinical benefit rate.

Evaluable disease only

a. Complete response (CR)
The disappearance of all known disease, determined by 2 observations not less than 4 weeks apart.

b. Partial response (PR)
Estimated decrease in tumor size of 50% or more determined by 2 observations not less than 4 weeks apart. In addition, there can be no appearance of new lesions or progression of any lesion.

c. Progressive disease (PD)
Estimated increase of 25% or more in existing lesions or appearance of new lesions.

d. No change (NC)
No significant changes for at least 4 weeks. This includes an estimated decrease of less than 50% and/or estimated increase of less than 25% of existing lesions.

RECIST criteria

Evaluation of tumor response is done for both target and non target lesions (see chapter XI.5).

Target lesions

a. Complete response (CR)
Disappearance of all target lesions.

b. Partial response (PR)
At least a 30% decrease in the sum of the longest diameter (LD) of target lesions taking as reference the baseline sum LD.

c. Progression (PD)
At least a 20% increase in the sum of LD of target lesions taking as references the smallest sum LD recorded since the treatment started or the appearance of one or more new lesions.

d. Stable disease (SD)
Neither sufficient shrinkage to qualify for PR nor sufficient increase to qualify for PD taking as references the smallest sum LD since the treatment started.

Confirmatory measurements
To be assigned a status of PR or CR, changes in tumor measurements must be confirmed by 2 observations not less than 4 weeks apart.

In case of SD measurements must have met the SD criteria at least once after study entry at a minimum interval (in general, not less than 6–8 weeks) that is defined in the protocol.

Non target lesions

a. Complete response (CR)
Disappearance of all non-target lesions and normalization of tumor marker level.

b. Incomplete response/Stable disease
Persistence of one or more non-target lesion(s) or/and maintenance of tumor marker level above the normal limits.

c. Progression (PD)
Appearance of one or more new lesions and/or unequivocal progression of existing non-target lesions. Although a clear progression of "non target" lesions only is exceptional, in such circumstances, the opinion of the treating physician should prevail and the progression status should be confirmed later on by the review panel (or study chair).

XI.5 Determination of overall response

WHO criteria

If measurable disease is present at different sites in a given patient, the result of each site should be recorded separately. The number of selected lesions per site should not exceed three and in all sites not more than five lesions must be selected. An overall assessment of response involves all sites.

In patients with measurable disease, the poorest response designation shall prevail. If in the totals of responses by organ site there are equal or greater numbers of complete plus partial responses than of "no change" designations, then overall response will be partial. If progressive disease exists in any lesion of sufficient size or when a new lesion appears, then the overall result will be "progressive disease". Mixed responses with a progressive site are considered progressive disease but the response per site must also be documented. The definition of complete response as overall response assumes the disappearance of all measurable and non-measurable lesions. Progression in non-measurable lesions should be taken to indicate progression regardless of what happens in measurable disease.

RECIST criteria

To assess objective response, it is necessary to estimate the overall tumor burden at baseline to which subsequent measurements will be compared. All measurable lesions up to a maximum of 5 lesions per organ and 10 lesions in total, representative of all involved organs, should be identified as target lesions and will be recorded and measured at baseline. Target lesions should be selected on the basis of their size (those with the longest diameter) and their suitability for accurate repetitive measurements (either by imaging techniques or clinically). A sum of the longest diameter (LD) for all target lesions will be calculated and reported as the baseline sum LD. The baseline sum LD will be used as reference by which to characterize the objective tumor response.

All other lesions (or sites of disease) should be identified as non-target lesions. Measurements are not required but the presence or absence of each should be noted throughout follow-up.

The determination of overall response takes into account the evaluation of target and non-target lesions and of the appearance of new lesions according to the following table.

Target lesions	Non target lesions	New lesions	Overall response
CR	CR	No	CR
CR	Incomplete response/SD	No	PR
PR	Non-PD	No	PR
SD	Non-PD	No	SD
PD	Any	Yes or no	PD
Any	PD	Yes or no	PD
Any	Any	Yes	PD

XI.6 Evaluation of bone metastases

For *bone metastasis* a separate set of criteria is necessary.

a.   Complete response (CR)
Complete disappearance of all lesions on X-ray or scan for at least 4 weeks.

b.   Partial response (PR)
Partial decrease in size of lytic lesions on X-ray, recalcification of lytic lesions for at least 4 weeks.

c.   Progressive disease (PD)
Increase in size of existing (lytic) lesions or appearance of new (lytic) lesions.

d.   No change (NC)
Because of the slow response of bone lesions the designation "no change" should not be applied until at least 8 weeks have passed from start of therapy.

N.B.: Occurrence of bone compression or fracture and its healing should not be used as the sole indicator for evaluation of therapy. Bone metastasis are considered non measurable lesions according to the RECIST criteria.

XI.7 Duration of response

WHO criteria

a. The duration of a complete response should last from the date the complete response was first recorded to the date progressive disease is first noted.
b. For patients who only achieve a partial response, only the period of overall response should be recorded. The period of overall response which is measured for all the responders (PR + CR) lasts from the first day of treatment to the date of first observation of progressive disease.

RECIST criteria

The duration of response is measured from the time measurement criteria are met for CR/PR (whichever is first recorded) until the first date that recurrent or progressive disease is objectively documented.

References

1. Response evaluation criteria in solid tumors (www3.cancer.gov/dip/RECIST.htm).
    See also:
    – Therasse P, Arbuck SG, Eisenhauer EA, Wanders J, Kaplan RS, Rubinstein L, Verweij J, Van Glabbeke M, van Oosterom AT, Christian MC, Gwyther SG. New guidelines to evaluate the response to treatment in solid tumors. European Organization for Research and Treatment of Cancer, National Cancer Institute of the United States, National Cancer Institute of Canada. *J Natl Cancer Inst.* 2000 Feb 2;92(3):205–16.
    – Therasse P. Measuring the clinical response. What does it mean? *Eur J Cancer.* 2002 Sep;38(14):1817–23.

XII. Systemic treatment

XII.1 Chemotherapy: standard criteria for dose reductions or delays in administration

XII.2 Endocrine therapy

XII.3 Bisphosphonate therapy

XII.4 Trastuzumab (Herceptin®) therapy

XII.1 Chemotherapy: standard criteria for dose reductions or delays in administration

a. Delay in start of treatment

If previous treatment has been chemotherapy, all toxic manifestations of that treatment must have disappeared; an interval of 3 weeks is recommended (or 6 weeks in the case of mitomycin C, nitrosureas or high dose chemotherapy).

In case of previous hormonal treatment (estrogens, antiestrogens, androgens, progestins) and a positive response, treatment should ideally be withdrawn for at least 4 weeks prior to start of cytostatics in order to exclude a withdrawal remission. However, this is frequently not possible (for both medical and psychological reasons), and therefore it is often not a practical consideration. The interval between date of progression and start of next treatment has to be specified in the protocol. Patients who had a failure on aromatase inhibitors can start immediately.

b. Dose modifications for phase III trials

The schedule of dose modifications should be specified in the protocol. In the first instance, treatment should be delayed rather than dose reduced. Delays should be minimised, especially in the adjuvant/neo-adjuvant setting, so that wherever possible patients should be retreated as soon as their counts recover, which may be only 2–3 days after the scheduled day. Dose reductions should be implemented only for repeated toxicity in the case of neutropenia, or in the case of severe toxicity (febrile neutropenia, grade III GI symptoms etc.). Grade IV neutropenia should not be an indication for a dose reduction, unless complicated by infection/sepsis or if it persists for 7 or more days. Each protocol should specify the precise rules for that particular study, but in general the following approach is recommended before each (half) cycle:

Dose % all drugs	Neutrophils[1]		White blood cells[1]		Platelets[1]	Other Grade III/IV
100%	>1	and	>2.5	and	>100	Absent
80%	>1	and	>2.5	and	>100	If recovered to Grade <2
Delay until recovery	>1	and/or	>2 & <3	and/or	>75–100	Absent
Delay until recovery	<1	and/or	<2	and/or	<75	Persists > Grade 1

[1] All values $\times\ 10^9$/l.

c. Postponement

If at the beginning of subsequent cycles the Neutrophil (Granulocyte) count is less than $1 \times 10^9/l$ (or if not available, total WBC is less than $2.5 \times 10^9/l$) and/or platelet count is less than $100 \times 10^9/l$, treatment is postponed until recovery (preferably 2–3 days). If myelosuppression persists for a week or more, the cycle should be started with dose reduced as indicated below:

Dose % all drugs	Neutrophils[1]		White blood cells[1]		Platelets[1]	Other Grade III/IV
100%	>1	and	>2.5	and	>100	Absent
80%	>1	and/or	>2 & <3	and/or	>75–100	If recovered
Delay until recovery	<1	and/or	<2	and/or	<75	Persists > Grade 1

[1] All values $\times 10^9/l$.

If postponement of therapy is necessary for more than three weeks, the patient goes off-study.

If any other grade III/IV toxicity occurs (with the exception of alopecia), then treatment should be delayed until it has improved to grade I or less. Thereafter treatment should be re-introduced at 80% of the initial dose.

If leukocyte and/or thrombocyte counts are too low to start the second part of a multi-part cycle (e.g. day 8 in classical/Bonadonna CMF), that particular cycle is considered as completed. In this situation the next cycle should start 21 days after start of the first part of that particular cycle.

- Kidney function: dose modification to be specified for the drug chosen.
- Liver function: dose modification to be specified for the drug chosen.
- In case of *phase II studies* leukocyte and thrombocyte counts will be specified in the protocol for that particular drug.

XII.2   Endocrine therapy

a.   Indications

Advanced disease:

- Disease that is known to be ER and/or PgR positive.
- ER and PgR unknown with indication of potential endocrine sensitivity.
  - Long disease free interval
  - Response to previous endocrine therapy
  - Absence of visceral disease
- In cases with rapid progression or extensive visceral involvement, treatment with chemotherapy is advisable.

Early disease:

- Following loco-regional curative therapy, if disease is known to be ER and/or PgR positive.
- Following loco-regional recurrence, even if excised/irradiated, consider if:
  - Known to be ER and/or PgR positive
  - Long disease free interval
  - Response to previous endocrine therapy

Her-2 positive breast cancer:

- Her-2 positivity is not a contra-indication to endocrine therapy, although the available data suggest that the probability of response to endocrine therapy may be lower.

b.   Choice of therapy

The choice of therapy depends on prior endocrine exposure:

- Women given adjuvant endocrine therapy are usually treated with a different agent upon recurrence, unless the disease recurred at least one year after stopping adjuvant endocrine therapy.
- There is no grade A evidence for any particular sequence of endocrine agents in post-menopausal women, and although the third generation aromatase agents have some advantages over tamoxifen in advanced disease, they are not yet standard therapy in the adjuvant setting.

Premenopausal patients:

- Tamoxifen is widely used, particularly in the adjuvant setting.
  - Although to date there is no level 1 evidence for its use following chemotherapy, extrapolation from other data suggests that it is highly likely to be effective.
  - Following chemotherapy, there is no level 1 evidence for using combined ovarian ablation and tamoxifen, although it is common practice

- Ovarian ablation (surgically or by radiotherapy) or medical suppression by an LHRH agonist.
  - In the adjuvant setting, ovarian ablation has been shown to be as effective as CMF chemotherapy alone for women with ER and/or PgR positive tumours
  - There are data suggesting that women who become post-menopausal following adjuvant chemotherapy may have a better outcome, whether this is due to the chemotherapy or the addition of an LHRH agonist
  - In advanced disease, LHRH agonist should preferentially be given in combination with tamoxifen

- If already treated with tamoxifen, LHRH agonists are often given with third generation aromatase inhibitors although there are no randomized trial data to confirm this approach.

Postmenopausal patients:

- tamoxifen (20 mg/day) remains standard of care for adjuvant therapy
  - if contra-indicated anastrazole is at least as effective and is associated with less thrombo-embolism
- in advanced disease, third generation aromatase inhibitors (anastrazole, letrozole and exemestane) are at least as effective as tamoxifen, and are often now given as first line therapy
- exemestane is active after non-steroidal aromatase inhibitors (anastrazole, letrozole) and is therefore often used upon progression
- faslodex appears to be equivalent to anastrazole after failure of tamoxifen, but its only advantage appears to be that it can be given by injection if compliance is a concern
- high-dose estrogens and progestogens remain options for later lines of therapy
- corticosteroids are rarely used now as an anti-cancer agent
- Osteoporosis (non-steroidal aromatase inhibitors, corticosteroids).

Minimal duration of therapy: 2 months.

c. Assessment of response

According to general rules (see Chapter X).

d. Specific side effects

- tumour flare (tamoxifen, estrogens, LHRH agonists)
- thromboembolic (tamoxifen, estrogens, progestins)
  - of the third generation aromatase inhibitors, only anastrazole has been shown to be associated with fewer thrombotic events than tamoxifen
- weight gain, depression (high doses of progestins, corticosteroids)
- hot flushes (LHRH agonists, tamoxifen, aromatase inhibitors)
- arthralgia (tamoxifen, aromatase inhibitors)

e. Additional remarks

- the predictive value of ER and *especially PgR* is probably optimal if the determination has been done before the start of endocrine therapy
- previous palliative chemotherapy does not exclude patients for subsequent endocrine therapy.
- there is no evidence of any advantage for giving chemotherapy and endocrine therapy cocurrently, and there are data in the adjuvant setting to suggest that this may be disadvantageous (higher rate of thrombosis and poorer disease-free survival).

XII.3   Bisphosphonate therapy

a.   Indications

It is clear from several studies that this class of agents can have a significant beneficial effect on the skeletal complications of metastastic breast cancer, including bone pain. Bisphosphonates are usually, but not invariably, given in combination with another anti-cancer agents. This is because although there are in vitro data to indicate that some members of this family can have direct anti-cancer effects, their primary clinical use is to reduce bone resorption and thus reduce the clinical consequences of bone metastases.

Advanced disease:

–   Metastatic breast cancer to bone.
  •   The absence of lytic disease is not a contra-indication, but many of the trials demon-strating the benefit of prophylactic bisphosphonates did require the presence of lytic disease
–   Hypercalcaemia of malignancy.

Early disease:

–   Currently NOT indicated in this setting other than in clinical trials, or for the treatment of osteoporosis.

b.   Choice of therapy

The choice is between oral therapy and intravenous therapy. The most convincing data for efficacy come from studies involving the second and third generation aminobisphosphonates.

–   *Oral.* Currently only the non-aminobisphosphonate clodronate is available.
–   *Intravenous.* There are three available agents (clodronate, pamidronate and zoledronate).

c.   Assessment of response

Objective assessment is difficult. The best measure of benefit is prevention or reduction of skeletal-related events (radiotherapy to bone, spinal cord compression, orthopaedic surgery, bone fractures, and hypercalcaemia).

d.   Specific side effects

–   RENAL FAILURE
  •   This is rare, particularly with the oral agents.
  •   Most commonly (in less than 5% of patients) this takes the form of a slow, not com-pletely reversible rise in serum creatinine.
  •   For intravenous bisphosphonates, the speed of infusion appears to relate to the risk of a significant rise in creatinine.
  •   Patients should have their serum creatinine monitored regularly during therapy, but it is not essential that the result is available before administration if the previous value was within the normal range

–   MINOR FLU LIKE REACTIONS
  •   These are common, and usually diminish with subsequent administrations
  •   They can be prevented with simple antipyretics such as paracetamol

- GASTRO-INTESTINAL SIDE EFFECTS
  - These are common, particularly with oral agents, but can also occur with the intra-venous preparations

e. *Frequency and duration of adminstration*

- The current license is for 4-weekly administration with the intravenous drugs, and daily for the oral agents.
- However, it is clear that this may not be optimal for all patients.
  - Studies are underway or proposed looking at tailoring both dose and frequency according to the biochemical effect of the drug on bone resorption
- The optimal duration of therapy is unknown.
  - The largest Phase III trials gave the drugs for up to 2 years, with in some cases increasing benefit seen during the second year, so that shorter administration is not recommended.
  - Many clinicians feel that continued therapy beyond 2 years is indicated in the absence of significant toxicity
  - There are NO randomized data currently available to confirm this.

XII.4   Trastuzumab (Herceptin®) therapy

a.   Indications

Advanced disease:

–   Disease that is known to be Her-2 positive (3+ by immunohistochemistry or FISH +ve).

Early disease:

–   Currently NOT indicated in this setting other than in clinical trials.

b.   Choice of therapy

The choice is between monotherapy and in combination with chemotherapy. However, the current clinical trial data strongly suggests that this drug is more effective if given in combination with a taxane.

–   *Monotherapy.* There is no clear data to point to a particular sequence of chemotherapy and Herceptin® when given as monotherapy. The drug is active when given as first-line therapy for advanced breast cancer, and as 2nd/3rd line.
–   *Combination.* The drug should not be given in combination with an anthracycline except within a carefully monitored clinical trial, due to the risk of cardiotoxicity. Two randomized trials (one only available to date in abstract form) suggest that there is evidence for synergy if Herceptin® is given in combination with a taxanes. Phase II data suggest that the same may be true with vinorelbine. Data with other chemotherapy agents are lacking.

c.   Cessation of therapy

–   Currently, most guidelines for the use of Herceptin® suggest that, in common with other anti-cancer agents, it should be stopped upon tumour progression.
–   However, significant anecdotal experience suggests that it can be continued in combination with a different chemotherapy agent with clinical benefit.

d.   Assessment of response

According to general rules (see Chapter XI).

e.   Specific side effects

–   CARDIAC FAILURE
    •   This is the commonest serious side effect, and the drug should only be given to patients with normal Left ventricular function (LVF).
    •   Patients should have their LVF assessed regularly during therapy, e.g. every 3 months, by either echocardiography or MUGA scan.
    •   The risk of cardiotoxicity is increased by prior anthracycline exposure, but can occur in patients without a history of use of these agents.

–   ANAPHYLAXIS
    •   This is rare, but is potentially life-threatening.
    •   The risk appears to be increased in patients with significant lung disease, in whom the drug should be used with caution.
    •   Of the third generation aromatase inhibitors, only anastrazole has been shown to be associated with fewer thrombotic events than tamoxifen

- MINOR FLU LIKE REACTIONS
  - These are common, and usually diminish with subsequent administrations
  - There is increasing evidence that there may be a slightly higher incidence of myelo-suppression when Herceptin® is given with chemotherapy.

f. Frequency of administration

- The current license is for weekly administration at the dose of 2 mg/Kg with a loading dose on the first week of 4 mg/Kg.
- An alternative 3-weekly schedule is available, with an 8 mg/Kg loading dose on the first cycle, and 6 mg/Kg every three weeks thereafter.
  - Phase II data suggests that this schedule in combination with taxol is as active as the weekly one.
  - No randomized data are currently available for the three-weekly schedule.
  - There is no evidence to date that either the three weekly schedule, nor a higher dose weekly schedule, are associated with any increase in serious or cardiac toxicity.
- Other loading schedules are being tested, but data are not yet available.

g. Other comments

- The half-life of this agent appears to be around 28 days, so that caution must be exercised in patients who are to receive an anthracycline after Herceptin®: current recommendations are to wait a few months before using any cardiotoxic drugs.

XIII.   Hereditary breast cancer

XIII. Hereditary breast cancer

Hereditary breast cancer may be considered when a family history suggests an autosomal dominant pattern of breast cancer inheritance. Features of such a family history include early age at diagnosis, multiple relatives with breast, or in some cases ovarian cancer, and more frequently bilateral breast cancer. It is estimated that 5–10% of all breast cancers may be attributable to hereditary breast cancer. By definition, familial breast cancer is classified as the index patient with carcinoma of the breast with one or more first- and/or second-degree relatives affected by breast cancer. The remainder of breast cancer cases, when no breast carcinomas among a patient's first- and second-degree relatives are present, are referred as sporadic cases. Because of low-penetrance genes, lack of information, small families and ignoring of extra-breast tumours, a clear distinction between familial, hereditary and sporadic breast cancer is not always possible.

Recent advances in molecular biology have enabled the identification of gene mutations, which are responsible for an increased risk of developing breast and other cancers. At present, several gene mutations are known to manifest in hereditary breast cancer: *BRCA1* on chromosome 17 and *BRCA2* on chromosome 13 in families with breast and/or ovarian cancer; *CHEK2**1100delC in families with breast and/or colon cancer. In addition, breast cancer may be a feature as part of a syndrome: *p53* in Li-Fraumeni syndrome; *PTEN* in Cowden syndrome; *STK11/LKB1* in Peutz-Jeghers syndrome; and *ATM* in ataxia telangiectasia. By contrast, ataxia telangiectasia is an autosomal recessive disorder. Male breast cancers are more frequently observed in *BRCA2*-mutation families, while family members with a *BRCA1*-mutation are associated with a higher lifetime risk of ovarian cancer. Other types of cancer than breast cancer are reported more frequently in syndromes, e.g. thyroid cancer in Cowden syndrome, and evidence suggests an increased risk of prostate cancer in male *BRCA1/2*-mutation carriers. Therefore, identification of these germline mutations by genetic testing enhance risk assessment of breast and other cancers in some families more accurately than in the past.

A family history should include both paternal and maternal sides of the family, healthy as well as affected relatives with all types of cancer, approximate ages at diagnosis and ages at death, if known. Table 1 lists the criteria for hereditary breast cancer, based on family history.

Table 1:   Family history risk criteria for Hereditary Breast/Ovarian cancer.

- breast cancer in ≥1 first degree relative ≤40 years or bilateral primary breast cancers of any age
- breast cancer in ≥2 relatives with breast cancer, with ≥1 diagnosed at age ≤50 years
- breast cancer in ≥1 relative and ovarian cancer in ≥1 relative
- ovarian cancer in ≥1 first-degree relative
- ovarian cancer in ≥2 relatives
- women or men with a blood relative with a known mutation in a breast cancer susceptibility gene

Women, who met one of the criteria, should be referred to a family cancer clinic. Also, women with a personal history of breast cancer ≤40 years and women aged ≤50 years at diagnosis with a family history of breast cancer should be referred for genetic counselling. In general, women from these families should be advised to undergo regular breast cancer surveillance. Recommendations include monthly breast self-examination, breast examination by a physician twice a year with an annual mammography and in case of a BRCA1/2-mutation-carrier breast magnetic resonance imaging. However, follow-up schemes differ and less frequent examinations are suggested by others.

Genetic testing (*BRCA1*, *BRCA2* and also *p53* gene mutations) should be considered. The chance of finding gene mutations is highest in affected members. DNA-testing in otherwise healthy women from suspected hereditary breast cancer families without the possibility of confirmation in affected members, i.e. DNA not available, carries the risk of finding polymorphisms not resulting in a malfunctionary gene (and hence with false suggestions).

Several sessions of pre- and post-test counselling are needed. Prevention decisions can extensively be discussed and compliance of surveillance may be higher if a gene mutation is identified. Some reassurance might come from a negative test result. However, if test results are negative, the risk still can be elevated; a fortiori the risk is unknown if tests are negative in the diseased family members. Insurance and possibly employment difficulties may arise after a positive test finding; also sensitive family issues may arise.

All these pros and cons should be discussed prior to a decision of testing. The best place for this exchange of information is the family cancer clinic.

It is unknown whether hormone replacement therapy (HRT) or other endocrine manipulation should be avoided in women with a possible genetic predisposition for breast cancer. A large case-control study observed a small increased risk of breast cancer among *BRCA1*-mutation carriers who used oral contraceptives before 1975, before 30 years of age and more than 5 years. It remains unclear whether *BRCA2*-mutation carriers have increased risks when using oral contraceptives. More recent studies showed an increased risk in postmenopausal women with long-time use of HRT. Therefore, in general practise the use of oral contraceptives in young women under age 30 years should be outweighed individually against the risks of unwanted pregnancies and other forms of contraception should be advised. In older, postmenopausal women from breast cancer families, the use of HRT should be discouraged.

Chemoprevention and/or prophylactic surgery should be discussed in very high risk cases. However, subgroup analysis with very small numbers failed to show a risk reduction in *BRCA1*-mutation carriers, whereas a risk reduction in *BRCA2*-mutation carriers was suggested. The possible effect of chemoprevention is further being tested in trial setting.

Prophylactic surgery is a major operation, especially psychologically. The counselling aspects are highly important. Removal of both breasts, eventually with a breast reconstruction, demonstrated a clear reduction in breast cancer incidence, although long-term follow-up and complications have to be monitored carefully. It must be emphasized that removal of all breast tissue is technically difficult and a very small chance of developing breast cancer might be uneventful. Also, removal of both ovaries (and Fallopian tubes) decreases the rate of developing breast cancer by 50% and ovarian cancer by more than 90%. Postoperative supplementation of HRT still remains a matter of debate and future studies have to evaluate its implications.

Centralization of such high-risk women is advisable to monitor complications and efficacy of the procedure.

XIV. Guidelines for assessing quality of life in EORTC breast studies

XIV.1 Selection of trials in which quality of life is relevant

Measurement of Quality of Life (QL) is not equally important in all clinical studies in breast cancer. The decision whether to measure QL should be based on the likely impact of the findings on recommendations for treatment once the study is completed, and should take into account resource implications. Many studies have failed to yield meaningful QL results because of poor compliance with completion of questionnaires resulting mainly from administrative failures in institutions and unwillingness of staff to administer questionnaires to ill patients. Therefore careful consideration should be given to feasibility before deciding to evaluate QL.

QL evaluation is rarely appropriate in Phase I and Phase II trials, but these trials may be used to pilot test QL questionnaires or in certain cases provide a hypothesis for future phase III trials. In addition, these trials may also allow an opportunity for researchers to gain experience in administering the instruments. In cases where no validated instruments are available, such early studies may allow researchers to gain some knowledge concerning the feasibility of using these measures with the given population. QL may also be measured in randomized Phase II studies that are expected to continue as Phase III trials in which QL is considered an important outcome measure.

In Phase III studies, QL measurement can be considered marginal when a small difference in QL and a substantial difference in survival are expected. It is considered central when a substantial effect on QL is expected and/or a small improvement in survival. Recent literature suggests that pre-treatment QL variables may have important prognostic significance for survival and response to treatment in advanced disease, and eventually they may be used for stratifying patients in clinical trials.

QL evaluation is likely to be particularly important in the following situations:

- A trial in which QL is the primary endpoint (e.g. the comparison of two palliative treatments)
- A trial in which no significant difference in disease-/progression-free survival or overall survival is expected between treatments (equivalence trial). In this situation treatment-associated morbidity will be of primary importance, and QL evaluation may provide important information for subsequent recommendations about treatment options.
- A trial with expected significant differences in outcome in which improvements are achieved at the expense of major toxicity (e.g. high dose chemotherapy plus bone marrow transplantation versus standard chemotherapy). In this situation QL considerations may be taken into account when recommending and deciding on treatment options.

A recent paper suggesting guidelines and a checklist for protocol writers and authors of QL studies wishing to assess QL in clinical trials has recently been published [1].

XIV.2   Relevant variables

QL as measured in cancer clinical trials is generally agreed to comprise a number of different "domains" that include physical, social and emotional function and symptoms. Although interviews are considered the "gold standard" for assessing individual QL, this method is not feasible in clinical trials, and so patient-completed questionnaires have been developed for this purpose. The EORTC QLQ-C30 core questionnaire is the instrument of choice in EORTC QL studies. This measure includes five function scales, several symptoms that commonly occur in cancer and "global" questions covering overall health and QL. There is also a specific breast cancer module (EORTC QLQ-BR23) that may be used to supplement the core questionnaire. The module contains questions relating to side effects of treatment (surgery, radiation therapy, chemotherapy and hormone therapy) and aspects of body image and sexuality. Both questionnaires have been validated and are reliable.

The choice of relevant variables will be dictated by the particular research question. Many studies that measure QL are exploratory in nature and are not designed to answer specific QL questions. For these studies the QLQ-C30 may be sufficient. However, optimally one should select specific QL endpoints *a priori* and design the study with sufficient power to answer the questions posed. In this case, specific items on the QLQ-C30 and/or QLQ-BR23 may be selected when designing the study. In addition, the EORTC Quality of Life Groups Item Bank provides an additional database of valid and reliable questions assessing all aspects of QL. This Item Bank allows additional study-specific questions to be added to existing questionnaires. Researchers wishing to use this should contact the EORTC Quality of Life Unit.

XIV.3   Design of the study

Most QL studies in the EORTC Breast Cancer Group will be undertaken in the context of randomized trials. This implies the comparison of treatment arms in which respondents are grouped on the basis of random selection. In such studies predictors of QL generally will be distributed equally between the treatment groups.

Information to assist in sample size calculations based on the QLQ-C30 may be found in the Reference Values Manual available from the EORTC Quality of Life Unit, EORTC Data Center, Brussels.

The number and frequency of measurements should be specified in the protocol and should be similar across all treatment arms. The schedule of measurements will depend on the study question, but will usually involve assessments before, during and after treatment. To reduce administrative burden and to optimize compliance, the minimum number of measurements should be used, and these should be timed to yield maximum information about changes in QL due to treatment and changing disease status.

There should be a baseline measurement before randomization at the start of treatment. This measurement is crucial and every effort should be made to maximize compliance with it. It allows pre-treatment comparison between study groups, is the basis for assessing change over time, and may allow for detection of systematic bias where follow-up data are missing Baseline measurements may also enable prognostic factor analyses to be conducted for outcomes such as survival and response to treatment.

Young et al. [2] provide detailed discussion on the timing of QL measurements during treatment. The timing will depend on the study question, and might involve measurements at points of expected maximum and minimum toxicity. Scheduling of measurements may be time-based (e.g. every 6 weeks), event-based (e.g. at the end of the third cycle of treatment) or a combination of the two. The timing of assessments after treatment will depend on whether short or long-term effects are to be measured. To eliminate bias, measurements should occur at equal times in each arm relative to randomization and not to the end of treatment. Some studies will optimally require QL assessments until death.

XIV.4 Data collection

Many studies with QL as an endpoint have yielded inconclusive findings because of insufficient data quality resulting from missing forms and missing items. Sometimes this has arisen from the perception that collection of QL data is optional or less important than collection of clinical and toxicity data. There is considerable evidence to suggest that missing QL data arise more commonly from administrative failures that from patient-associated factors. If QL is considered an important endpoint of the study then careful attention should be paid to training those who administer questionnaires to understand the importance of collecting good quality data even when patients are ill. It should be the patient's decision to refuse to complete a questionnaire rather than staff taking a decision not to offer it when the patient is unwell. Monitoring of data quality during the trial should also be considered, with a named contact person responsible for collection of QL data at each participating institution.

Questionnaires may be administered in person during a clinic visit or by mail to the patient's home address. It is preferable for patients to complete the questionnaire in person in the clinic as it improves compliance, ensures that the data is provided at the appropriate time-point by the patient and not by a proxy, and allows checking for missing data so that omissions can be rectified (or documented with reasons given).

The timing of data collection is important. Baseline data collection is now mandatory in EORTC trials where QL is assessed, and should be collected before randomization. This ensures high levels of compliance and also that the outcome of randomization cannot influence any responses. In order to minimize all sources of potential bias it is recommended that the patient complete the questionnaire before seeing the physician.

Young et al. [2] provide a detailed discussion of practical issues relating to data collection, including optimizing compliance, the mode and time of delivery of questionnaires, proxy ratings and how to handle missing data. Bottomley et al. [3] provide details on recent approaches adopted within the EORTC on improving QL trials. Both documents are available from the EORTC Quality of Life Unit.

XIV.5 Analysis of the data (and report)

Analysis and interpretation of QL data are not straightforward, and both are areas of active research at present. At present the interpretation of findings pertaining to QL is uncertain, as it is generally not known whether statistical significance indicates clinical significance. Research is underway to determine the clinical significance of changes in EORTC QLQ-C30 scores. The EORTC QL Study Group has published a Reference Manual (Fayers et al. [4,5]) containing baseline QLQ-C30 scores for patients enrolled in cancer clinical trials to aid interpretation both of baseline data and changes over time. Practical guidelines for reporting results of QL assessments in clinical trials are available in Efficace et al. [1].

References

1. Efficace F, Bottomley A, Osoba D, Gotay C, Flechtner H, D'haese S, Zurlo A. Beyond the Development of Health-Related Quality-of-Life (HRQOL) Measures: A Checklist for Evaluating HRQOL Outcomes in Cancer Clinical Trials – Does HRQOL Evaluation in Prostate Cancer Research Inform Clinical Decision Making? *J Clin Oncol.* 2003 Sep 15;21(18):3502–11.
2. Young T, de Haes H, Fayers P, Brandberg E, Vanvoorden V, Bottomley A. Guidelines for assessing quality of life in clinical trials. EORTC Quality of Life Study Group Publications, Brussels. 2nd Edition, ISBN 2-930064-17, March 2002.
3. Bottomley A, Vanvoorden V, Flechtner H, Therasse P. The challenge and achievements of implementation of Quality of Life Research in cancer clinical trials. On behalf of the EORTC Quality of Life Group and EORTC Data Center. *European Journal of Cancer,* 39, 275–285, 2003.
4. Fayers P, Weeden S, Curran D. on behalf of the EORTC Quality of Life Study Group. EORTC QLQ-C30, Reference Values. EORTC Quality of Life Study Group. Brussels. 1998. ISBN 2-930064-11-0.
5. Fayers P, Aaronson N, Bjordal K, Groenvold M, Curran D, Bottomley A. EORTC QLQ-C30, Scoring Manual. 3rd Edition, EORTC Publications, Brussels. ISBN 2-9300 64-22-6, January 2001.

XV. Guidelines for the conduct of clinical trials within the EORTC Breast Cancer Group

XV.1 Responsibilities of the study coordinator

The Study Coordinator (SC) is responsible for all medical aspects related to the study and for its conduct. In this respect he will work closely with the Data Manager (DM), the Statistician and the Coordinating Physician at the Data Center (DC) during the entire course of the study.

The SC is responsible for the development of the protocol. After approval by the Data Center, the SC will submit the protocol to the EORTC Protocol Review Committee (PRC) according to the guidelines given on the EORTC internet homepage: www.eortc.be.

Before the start of the trial the SC will make sure that the case report forms (CRFs) to be used are properly adapted to the trial, preferably by testing them on a few patients. Soon after initiation of the trial (i.e. after enrolment of about 10% of the total patient population), the SC should review, together with the DM, the data for these patients. In this way any potential misunderstandings related to the protocol, the forms or the trial design could be detected at an early point in time. During the conduct of the clinical trial the SC has the following responsibilities:

- Trial Monitoring: Soon after the start of the study, the SC should visit the DC to determine patient accrual, review the data for the patients entered, evaluate patient eligibility, and discuss the problems encountered in the study with the Data Center staff. Where appropriate, quality control site visits to the participating institutions should be planned in conjunction with the Quality Assurance Unit of the Data Center.
- Preparation for group meetings: The DM will send a standard report of the study to the SC at least one week before the meeting. The SC will then check the tables and request additional information if necessary. The SC will present the data of his study at the meetings and discuss the status and the results with the group.
- Reporting trial results: The SC will prepare an abstract of the trial results for the important Oncology Meetings (EBCC, St. Gallen Breast Cancer Symposium, San Antonio Breast Cancer Symposium, ASCO, AACR, ESMO, ECCO, ESSO, ESTRO). He will also prepare the full publication of the trial or designate a co-investigator for that purpose, in order to submit the paper to a peer-review journal (preferably the European Journal of Cancer, the official EORTC journal) within 6 months of receiving the final analysis from the statistician.

XV.2 Responsibilities of the data manager at the Data Center

Before the start of the trial:

- Insure that all the necessary administrative formalities have been taken care of before activation of a study (PRC approval, trial insurance, regulatory approval) and allowing an institution to enter patients (investigator commitment statement, local ethics committee approval, normal lab values, investigator's CV, list of staff authorized to sign the case report forms).
- In collaboration with the SC the statistician and the coordinating physician design the CRFs for data collection and the eligibility checklist.
- Circulate a copy of the forms and the eligibility checklist to the participating centers.

Soon after the start of patient entry:

- Make sure the SC has made arrangements to review the data in due time for the first patients entered.
- Check that the forms are sent to the DC according to the schedule given in the protocol.

During the trial:

- Clarify with the investigators any data that are missing or seem unreliable.
- Inform the SC about any life threatening toxicity that may be reported.
- Remind the investigators to send the follow-up forms in due time. Once every 3 months compile a list of missing and overdue forms based on the Data Center's standard operating procedure for data timeliness.
- Prepare the semi-annual report on ongoing trials with the help of the SC, statistician, and coordinating physician.

At the end of the trial:

- Assist the SC in getting missing data.
- Assist the SC and the statistician in doing the final analysis.

XV.3 Responsibilities of individual investigators

- Provide the DM with the necessary documents (see XV.2) so that his center may be authorized to enter patients in the study.
- Send in the case report forms in due time.
- Report any serious adverse events according to the procedure described in the protocol.
- Give a prompt answer to the inquiries of the DM and/or the study coordinator.
- Be available and ready for site visits and prepare all the necessary documents for this purpose.

XV.4 Design of clinical trials

XV.4.1 Planning and preparation of a new trial

a. Administrative aspects

During the planning of a new study the DC team (data manager, statistician and coordinating physician of the group) must be involved with the design of the trial from the earliest possible moment. After general agreement on the objectives of the trial within the group, the team must critically review the first draft of the outline proposal of the protocol prepared by the SC, with special attention being paid to the:

- objectives of the trial (endpoints)
- patient selection criteria
- trial design and schema
- criteria of evaluation, definition of end points
- statistical considerations (prognostic/stratification factors, sample size, interim analyses, trial feasibility).

The team must approve the outline proposal before its submission to PRC. The statistician coordinates the development of the outline protocol.

The DC team must also review and approve the final version of the full protocol *before* its submission to the PRC.

After written notification of approval of the protocol by the PRC, the team must review the final version of the protocol, the first draft of the forms and the registration/randomization questions. The team must give its approval prior to their submission to the Form Review Committee (FRC). The data manager coordinates the development of Case Report Forms (CRF's).

b. Statistical aspects phase II trials

Stratification factors
In general, none except institution, unless each stratum is considered to be a study in itself.

Sample size
There is no universally accepted standard for calculating the number of patients required, although 2 stage trial designs are generally employed to allow for early termination due to lack of activity of the tested drug. Randomized phase II trials should be considered to test for simultaneous screening of new single agents or investigate new combination regimen with a standard control arm. In all cases the probability of rejecting an effective drug from further study should not be greater than 0.05. Two stage Simon optimal or minimax designs are often employed, or their extension by Bryant and Day to incorporate early stopping for toxicity. Other two stage designs that may be considered are the Gehan design for early phase II trials, the ECOG design, the Fleming two stage design and the sequential design (phase II-III).

c. Statistical aspects phase III trials

Stratification factors
All trials should be stratified by institution and by the most important prognostic factors. Because minimization is used to allocate treatments, several stratification factors may eventually be taken into account. It is recommended, however, to keep the randomization procedure simple by limiting the number of stratification factors to the 1 or 2 most important variables.

For adjuvant studies the following factors should generally be considered for stratification at entry on study: nodal status, menopausal status and hormone receptor status.

For studies in advanced disease the following factors should be considered for stratification at entry: performance status, presence of visceral metastases and hormone receptor status.

Trial end points and sample size

The first step is to determine the primary end point of the trial and the statistical analysis methods that will be used. Is the trial testing for equivalence or is a difference being sought? Will a one-sided or two-sided test be employed? In general, two-sided tests are to be preferred with error rates no larger than alpha = 0.05 and beta = 0.20.

In trials where time to event (duration of survival or progression free survival) is the main end point, the power to detect differences depends on the number of events that are observed, not on the number of patients entered. The number of events should be calculated based on the event rate in the control group, a *realistic* estimate of the size of the difference to be detected, whether a one- or two-sided test will be used and the size of the type I and type II errors, alpha and beta. The sample size is then calculated taking into account the duration of patient entry and the duration of follow-up after the last patient has been entered. Contrary to the number of events, the sample size is not unique. It is important that a sufficient number of patients be entered and followed for a sufficiently long period of time in order to observe the required number of events.

Realistic estimates of the expected accrual rate and duration of patient entry must be provided. In general, the expected duration of patient entry should *not* exceed 5 years.

Trials comparing more than two treatments are not very efficient and are generally not to be recommended. The exception are trials based on a 2 × 2 factorial design which in some cases may allow two questions to be asked without increasing the sample size.

d. Definition of end points phase II trials

Response to treatment

To be assessed in accordance with the guidelines given in chapter X and XI of this manual. The denominator of the response rate must at least include all eligible patients.

Because many new anticancer agents will not operate as cytotoxic but as cytostatic, other endpoints such as the clinical benefit or time to progression as defined below could also be considered. The determination of the clinical benefit rate includes all patients with complete response, partial response and stable disease. A meaningful duration of stable disease has to be a priori defined in the protocol and should last usually at least for 26 weeks after the start of treatment.

e. Definition of end points phase III trials

In the definitions which follow, disease "progression" will be understood to mean progression, relapse or recurrence as appropriate. Thus no distinction will be made between progression, relapse or recurrence when defining the following intervals of time.

Response to treatment

To be assessed in accordance with the guidelines given in chapter X and XI of this manual. The denominator of the response rate must at least include all eligible patients. Response assessment can seldom be a sufficient primary endpoint and should be considered with another measure of efficacy such as the quality of life or symptom control.

Time to progression (usually advanced disease)
Time to progression is calculated as the time interval between the date of randomization and the date of disease progression (see X.5). The denominator should include all patients.

In the case that the end point of interest has not yet been observed, then the end point is censored at the date of the last examination.

Progression free survival (usually advanced disease)
Progression free survival is calculated as the time interval between the date of randomization and the date of disease progression or death, whichever comes first (see X.5). If neither event has been observed, then it is censored at the date of the last follow up examination. The denominator should include all patients.

Disease-free interval (usually primary treatment and adjuvant trials)
The time interval between the date of randomization and the date of disease progression. For patients who die prior to progression, their follow-up is censored at the date of death. Otherwise it is censored at the date of the last follow-up examination. Note: use of the date of operation as starting point may yield a biased analysis if not all patients are operated at the same point in time (see also X.5).

Disease-free survival (usually primary treatment and adjuvant trials)
The time interval between the date of randomization and the date of disease progression or death, whichever comes first. If neither event has been observed, then it is censored at the date of the last follow-up examination. Note: use of the date of operation as starting point may yield a biased analysis if not all patients are operated at the same point in time (see also X.5).

Duration of survival
The time interval between the date of randomization and the date of death. Patients who are still alive are censored at the date of last follow-up. While a separate analysis of death due to malignant disease may be carried out (deaths due to other causes are censored at the date of death), the main analysis should include deaths due to any cause.

XV.4.2   Inclusion/exclusion of patients from analyses

Definitions

Eligibility: a patient is eligible if he/she meets all the patient inclusion criteria as defined in the protocol. Eligibility is based only on the patient's status at the time of entry in the trial and *cannot* be based on something that happens to the patient after registration or randomization. Patients thought by the data manager to be ineligible should be reviewed by the study coordinator as soon as possible.

Patients are no longer categorized as being "evaluable" or "not evaluable" (and thus no definition of "evaluable" is provided), but specific types of protocol violations are requested on the evaluation form filled out by the Study Coordinator.

Each patient will be reviewed by the Study Coordinator to determine if the patient was eligible and was treated and assessed in accordance with the protocol.

In trials which assess the response to treatment, the response to treatment must be filled out for *all randomized* patients, even for those patients who were ineligible or had major protocol violations.

Exclusion of patients from analyses

All patients registered or randomized in a trial must be accounted for. The number of patients entered and the number of eligible patients must be provided by treatment group. Reasons of ineligibility and reasons for the exclusion of eligible patients from the analysis must be given.

Analysis of response to treatment (phase II/phase III trials).

When response to treatment is an end point, all patients must be assessed for response whenever possible, even if there are major protocol treatment violations. An incorrect treatment schedule or administration, while noted on the evaluation form, is *not* an automatic cause of exclusion in the analysis of the response rate. Patients should be assigned one of the following categories:

a. complete response
b. partial response
c. stable disease
d. progression
e. unknown, not assessable for response

This last category includes patients who could not be assessed for response for any reason, for example patients who die or are lost to follow-up prior to assessment as defined in the protocol. The main analysis of the response rate should be done in all eligible patients counting patients in response categories d. and e. as treatment failures (progression). Subgroup analyses may sometimes be done where patients who have major protocol violations are excluded from the analysis of response to treatment. However, these subgroup analyses may *not* serve as the basis for drawing conclusions concerning treatment activity.

Phase II trials
Results must be provided in accordance with the above criteria.

Phase III trials
All randomized patients, *including ineligible ones*, must be treated and followed in accordance with the protocol whenever possible. If the cause of ineligibility is such that a patient cannot be kept in the protocol, then the patient must at least be followed for the duration of survival. Thus *all* patients, including ineligible ones, must be followed for survival.

In primary treatment, adjuvant and advanced studies, patients should be analyzed according to the "intent to treat" principle: all conclusions must be based on *all* randomized patients and according to the treatment group assigned by randomization.

Patients who are randomized and refuse all treatment must still be followed at least for the duration of survival. Patients who are randomized to one treatment and then for whatever reason receive one of the other protocol treatments will be analyzed as follows:

a. For analyses of treatment efficacy, the main analysis and all conclusions will be based on keeping the patient in the treatment group assigned by randomization.
b. For analyses of toxicity, analyses will be based on the treatment the patient actually received.

If more than 10% of the patients entered are ineligible, an analysis including only the eligible patients may also be carried out. Patients who are found to be "ineligible" based on an assessment, which is made after the start of protocol treatment, are *not* ineligible. They are to be considered as treatment failures and must continue to be followed for the duration of survival. Patients who do not meet the entry criteria based on histological review (or any other material which is taken *prior* to entry in the trial), but for which the conclusions are known only after the patient has been entered, are to be considered as ineligible. These patients should, however, continue to be followed in accordance with the protocol whenever possible.

XV.4.3   Interim analyses

Phase II trials

Early stopping rules
An early stopping rule in case of drug inactivity is to be written into the statistical considerations of the protocol. The Simon optimal 2 stage design is recommended.

Presentation of results
Data will be presented at the group meeting by the study coordinator on the basis of the last Data Center report.

Quality control
Data will be checked by the Data Manager DM before each update of the computer file. Dubious data will be discussed immediately with the Study Coordinator (SC). The SC will review complete files at the time of patient evaluation. If a program of site visits is implemented, the DM should be involved.

Phase III trials

During the period of patient entry, interim statistical analyses may be done in order to ensure that it is still ethical to continue patient entry. It should be specified in the protocol if interim statistical analyses are to be carried out while a trial is still open to entry.

The results of any interim analysis comparing treatment efficacy may not be presented to any of the participants of the trial as long as patients are still being entered. When interim statistical analyses are foreseen in the protocol, Independent Data Monitoring Committee (IDMC) should be appointed to monitor the study and evaluate the results of the interim analysis, taking individual as well as collective ethics and the results from other trials into consideration. The committee may decide to recommend closure of the trial or to amend the protocol. However, the final decision to close the trial or to amend the protocol is the responsibility of the SC and the group.

Early stopping rules
Conservative significance levels should be used so that the final analysis can be carried out at close to the usual 5% level of significance. It is recommended that only one endpoint, preferably a comparison of the duration of survival based on the logrank test, be used for early stopping. An alpha spending function based on the O'Brien-Fleming design, or Peto's plan whereby the trial is stopped early only if $P < 0.001$, are to be preferred for efficacy comparisons. For toxicity comparisons the O'Brien-Fleming design is quite conservative and the Pocock design may be considered.

Frequency
As requested by the IDMC.

Quality control
The statistician and DM should define the cross checks to be carried out by computer prior to the statistical analysis. All interim analyses of the primary end-points should include basic quality control checks: distribution of patient characteristics by treatment, distribution of important time intervals, and checks for possible inconsistencies not included in the original cross-checks.

XV.4.4   Final analysis

Phase II trials

Quality control
See XV.4.3 interim analyses.

Main endpoints
The endpoints that will be analyzed should be defined in the protocol as primary endpoints. These can include: response to treatment, time to progression, clinical benefit and side effects. A separate analysis could be carried out (if relevant and meaningful) for each level of any stratification factor that has been defined.

Phase III trials

Quality control
All previous quality control checks will be repeated at the time of the final analysis. Special attention will be paid to the distribution of date differences and data pertaining to the end points under study.

In order to assess the quality of institutional results, separate analyses may be carried out by institution when appropriate and feasible. Attention should be paid to the distribution of ineligible patients/protocol violations by institution and by treatment group as indicated on the patient evaluation form.

Main endpoints
Treatments will be compared according to the endpoints listed in the protocol using accepted statistical techniques:

- Time-to-event data (duration of survival, progression free survival, disease free interval): estimation of time to event is performed using the Kaplan-Meier technique and comparison by the log rank test.
- Categorical data (response to treatment, toxicity) is performed using the chi square test and chi square test for linear trend.

Results will be analyzed using the intent-to-treatment principle (all randomized patients). Analyses of endpoints according to the percentage of drug received or based on any other event occurring after entry on study (such as response) are, by definition, biased and are to be avoided when drawing conclusions.

It is important that any imbalances in the distribution of patient characteristics for very important prognostic factors (not used as prospective stratification factors) are taken into account by means of retrospective stratification.

Prognostic factors
The most important prognostic factors should be identified in a multivariate model (Cox proportional hazard) and the treatment comparisons adjusted retrospectively for any imbalances in these factors.

XV.5 Publication of results

The statistician should provide and discuss with the SC the statistical results of the trial. He/she should provide a written description of the statistical methods used and a summary of the results for inclusion in the final publication.

The Data Center team should review all texts and abstracts prior to their submission for publication or presentation, be included as co-authors in all paper and abstracts, and review the order and criteria for authorship. It is recommended to list all participating institutions in the acknowledgements section along with any sponsor that supported the study (including the US NCI).

The publication policy of the EORTC (Policy 009 available from www.eortc.be) should always apply.

XV.6   Authorship

All group presentations and publications must mention the EORTC in the title a
approved by the SC, group chairman and the DC team.

Authorship includes:

- the study coordinator (usually the first author)
- representative(s) of the member institutions which have contributed at least 10% of the
  eligible patients (members contributing less than 10% of patients may be included as
  co-authors at the discretion of the SC)
- two EORTC representatives of the data center team (statistician and coordinating
  physician)

Abstracts and draft publications must also be sent in advance to all co-authors and the
secretary and chairman of the group for their approval.

Publications in cooperation with other EORTC groups or other organizations will follow the
same rules and must meet the criteria of all participating groups.

·elopment process

.(Group, new ideas are first discussed in the Steering Committee,
.easibility, scientific content and interest from major centers (represented
ittee). Next a preliminary two page outline is discussed during the protocol
.on as to their scientific interest, practical feasibility and potential accrual.

ρproves the idea, the SC in conjunction with the EORTC DC develops an outline
.ter DC approval it is submitted to the PRC in accordance with the guidelines and
.t given on the EORTC internet homepage: www.eortc.be

.s concept is approved by the PRC, the full protocol is developed by a protocol writing
,mmittee within the group in conjunction with the DC. Once approved by the group and the
ᴐC it is submitted to PRC for final approval.

XV.6 Authorship

All group presentations and publications must mention the EORTC in the title and be approved by the SC, group chairman and the DC team.

Authorship includes:

- the study coordinator (usually the first author)
- representative(s) of the member institutions which have contributed at least 10% of the eligible patients (members contributing less than 10% of patients may be included as co-authors at the discretion of the SC)
- two EORTC representatives of the data center team (statistician and coordinating physician)

Abstracts and draft publications must also be sent in advance to all co-authors and the secretary and chairman of the group for their approval.

Publications in cooperation with other EORTC groups or other organizations will follow the same rules and must meet the criteria of all participating groups.

XV.7   Protocol development process

Within the EORTC Breast Group, new ideas are first discussed in the Steering Committee, particularly to check on feasibility, scientific content and interest from major centers (represented in the Steering Committee). Next a preliminary two page outline is discussed during the protocol development session as to their scientific interest, practical feasibility and potential accrual.

If the group approves the idea, the SC in conjunction with the EORTC DC develops an outline proposal. After DC approval it is submitted to the PRC in accordance with the guidelines and the format given on the EORTC internet homepage: www.eortc.be

If this concept is approved by the PRC, the full protocol is developed by a protocol writing committee within the group in conjunction with the DC. Once approved by the group and the DC it is submitted to PRC for final approval.